# DAUGHTER - i4U

And a woman was there who had been subject to bleeding for twelve years. She had suffered a great deal under the care of many doctors and had spent all she had, yet instead of getting better she grew worse. When she heard about Jesus, she came up behind him in the crowd and touched his cloak, because she thought, "If I just touch his clothes, I will be healed." Immediately her bleeding stopped and she felt in her body that she was freed from her suffering.

At once Jesus realized that power had gone out from him. He turned around in the crowd and asked, "Who touched my clothes?" "You see the people crowding against you," his disciples answered, "and yet you can ask, 'Who touched me?' " But Jesus kept looking around to see who had done it. Then the woman, knowing what had happened to her, came and fell at his feet and, trembling with fear, told him the whole truth. He said to her, "Daughter, your faith has healed you. Go in peace and be freed from your suffering."

## This Book is recommended for all Daughters

Forty percent of gynecological complaints by teen girls, young women & older women include complaints about disorders of the menstrual cycle

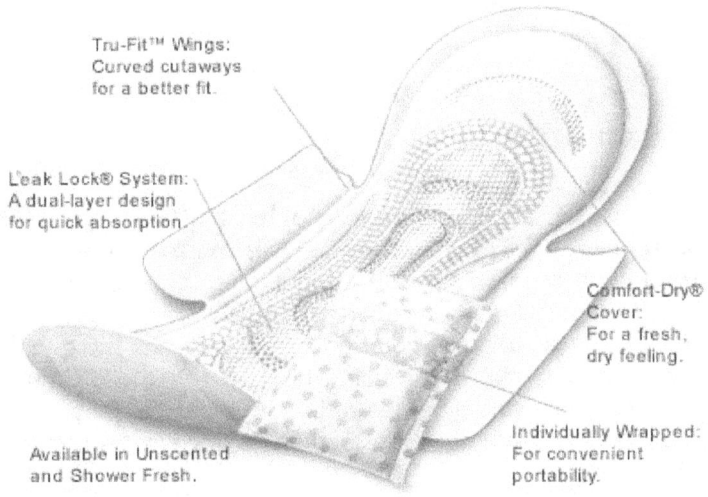

The Menstrual Cycle has Power to influence the performance of a DAUGHTER at School and in the workplace

*i4U*

© KCM 2018

**ALL RIGHTS RESERVED.**

No part of this publication may be used or reproduced in any manner whatsoever without written permission except for that provided for by the publisher.

The Author and the publisher disclaim responsibility for any adverse effects resulting directly or indirectly from suggested procedures, from undetected errors, or from the reader's misunderstanding of the text.

Furthermore, the Author and publisher do not accept responsibility from emotional or other damages caused by copying or imitation of actions demonstrated in this book.

## Acknowledgements

I sincerely acknowledge the permission granted to me by the **Royal College of Obstetricians and Gynaecologists (RCOG) to reproduce twelve patient information leaflets for this menstrual diary.** The RCOG produces guidelines as an educational aid to good clinical practice. They present recognised methods and techniques of clinical practice, based on published evidence, for consideration by obstetricians and gynaecologists and other relevant health professionals. This means that RCOG guidelines are unlike protocols or guidelines issued by employers, as they are not intended to be prescriptive directions defining a single course of management.

I also wish to acknowledge; Mrs. Morgan for sharing constructive thoughts and piloting this book & encouragement to roll it out to all Daughters in College, University, Workplace and in the Home country wide;

Ms. Kapalu for sharing her insights and an inspiring story about her amazing heroine, her niece, who rescued a Girl Child in grade eight; Seeing her classmate's uniform had been soiled, she told the boys in her class the headmaster wanted to see them at once. When the boys left the classroom, she and her friends came to the Aid of their classmate, saving her from an indelible scar of being laughed at and ridiculed by boys in class; Ms Gillian Gideon for believing in this little book and kept the original manuscript to this book for seven years before it was published. Including many I cannot list individually. This little Menstrual Information Diary is a fruition of your inspiring words.

# DEDICATION

This Information Menstrual Care Diary is dedicated to

All Daughters

It is also dedicated to

The Girl Child

# INTRODUCTION

The Menstrual Cycle is the most amazing phenomenon in the life of a Woman. Its beginning, referred to as Menarche, announces monumental changes in the life of a girl child. Its end, referred to as Menopause, ushers in other monumental changes in the lives of many Daughters. Some of these changes are so intense that they can alter the daughter's personality. This can affect her social functioning beginning at home and work place.

Daughters need special care to aid them stay afloat the hormonal storm raging inside their bodies. Everyone expects the young woman to hurriedly learn to manage herself and navigate the complex world around her. She is often judged harshly when she stumbles and falls.

**The menstrual cycle causes her to lose blood every Month. This may cause her Anemia, a medical condition that is characterized by; poor concentration, headaches, dizziness, weakness, getting tired easily, reduced mental capacity, low immunity, poor wound healing, poor appetite, lethargy, fainting, heart failure, poor oxygen delivery to body organs, poor skin health & poor performance in her daily errands.**

The Menstrual Cycle is intricately tied to Women's Health in Everyday Life; its understanding, monthly vigilance & management, is often critical if a young woman is to Enjoy Good Health in Everyday Life.

This *i4U*-Menstrual Care Diary is designed to assist Daughters of all age groups, record the ever changing information in their cycle. It is intended to generate interest among women to re examine this powerful phenomenon that continues to influence their lives and those around them even long after it is gone.

# Contents

- Example on how to use Your Diary — 9
1. January — 12
   i4U-PMS — 17
2. February — 25
   i4U- Pelvic Pain — 30
3. March — 36
   i4U- Early Miscarriage — 40
4. April — 49
   i4U-Caesarean Birth — 53
5. May — 62
   i4U-Ovarian Cysts — 66
6. June — 74
   i4U- Ovarian Cancer — 78
7. July — 88
   i4U- PID — 92
8. August — 103
   i4U- Birth Injury — 107
9. September — 114
   i4U- PE — 118

*i4U*

| | | |
|---|---|---|
| 10. | October | 124 |
| | *i4U*-Your Baby's movements in pregnancy | 128 |
| 11. | November | 135 |
| | *i4U*-Treatment for the Menopause | 139 |
| 12. | December | 150 |
| | *i4U*- The Vulva | 154 |

# Example

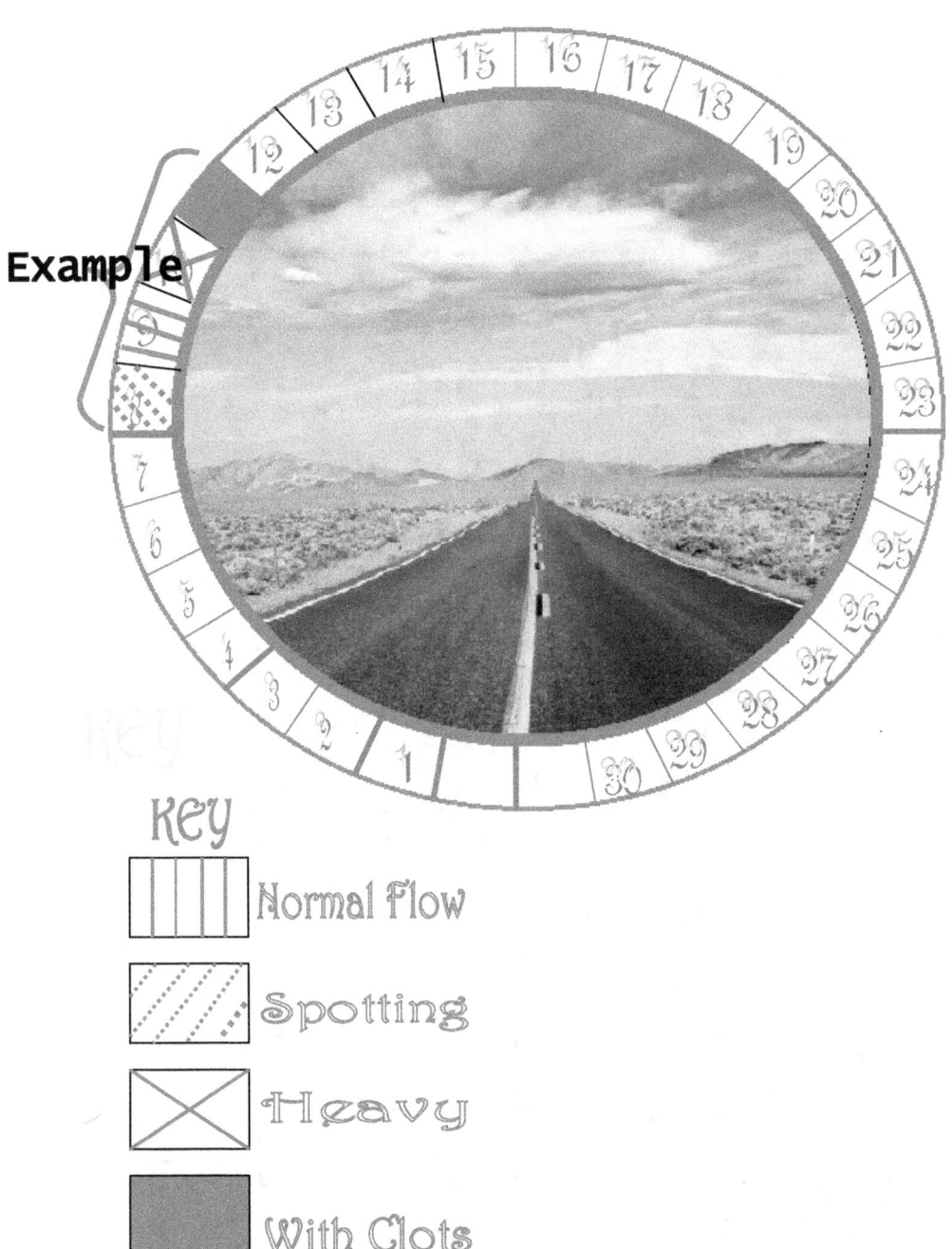

**Example**

### Key

| | |
|---|---|
| ||||| | Normal Flow |
| ▨ | Spotting |
| ⊠ | Heavy |
| ■ | With Clots |

*i4U*

- The Average duration of normal Menses is 3 – 7 days
- The length of a normal cycle is between 21 to 35 days
- The normal Blood Loss per cycle ranges between 13 to 80 milliliters
- A Soaked standard Pad or Tampon absorbs 5 to 15 milliliters of blood

This information could be used to estimate blood loss per cycle. To do this, complete the Sanitary Table for each month as shown below

| Day of Menses | # of Standard Pads / Number of Tampons used | | Improvised Pads used |
|---|---|---|---|
| | SOAKED (x) | NOT SOAKED (y) | |
| Day 1 | | 2 pads | 0 |
| Day 2 | 1 pad | 3 tampons | 0 |
| Day 3 | 3 tampons | 1 pad | 0 |
| Day 4 | 3 pads | 1 pad | 0 |
| Day 5 | | 2 tampons | 0 |
| Day 6 | | | |
| Day 7 | | | |

|  |  |  |  |
|---|---|---|---|
| TOTAL | 7 | 9 | 0 |
|  |  |  |  |

In the following pages, you can now follow your cycle and consult your doctor for medical advice whenever the cycle causes you concern. **You can also use this Diary to record your family planning information in a given month and document the side effects you notice.**

i4U

January 20......

wHeEL

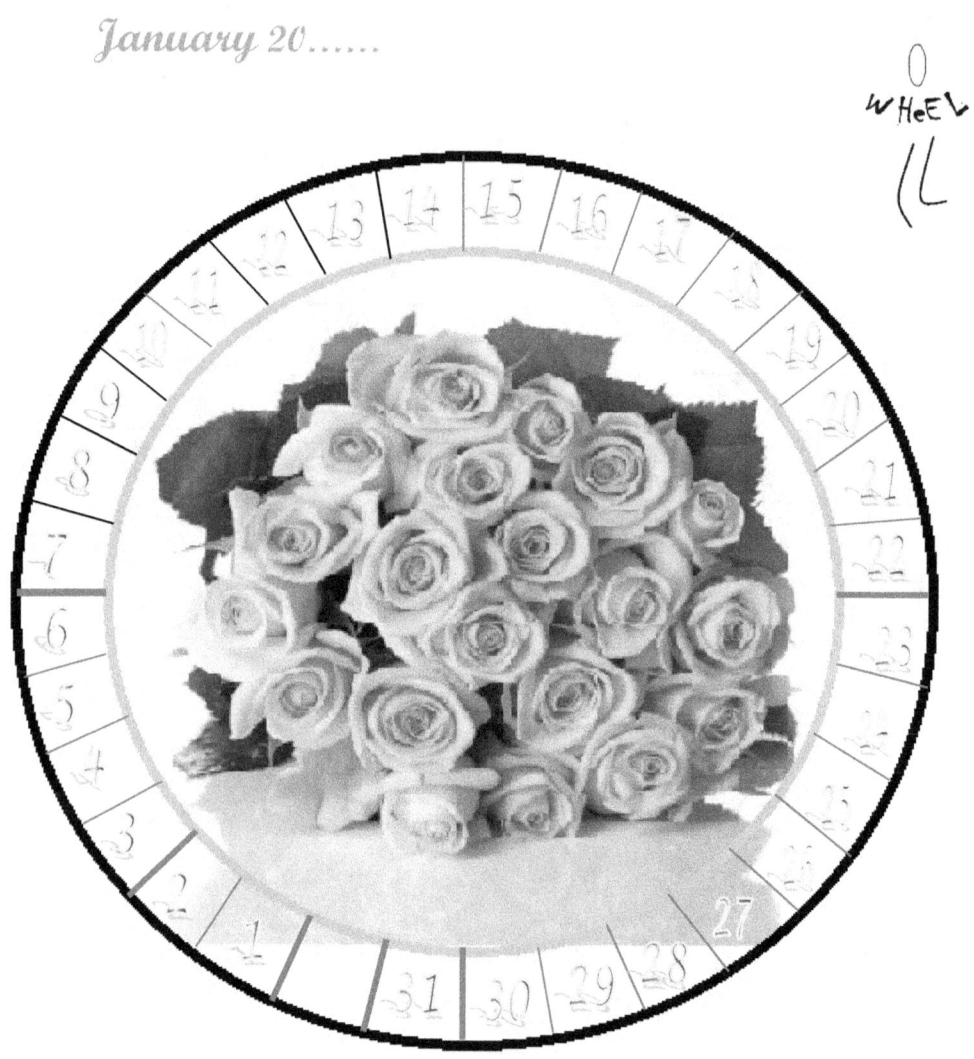

In the January Menstrual Cycle ( Tick were appropriate )

1) Period lasted longer than seven days     YES.... NO...
2) Used more pads than is usual for me      YES... NO...

3) Used more tampons than is usual for me YES...NO...
4) I Bled with Clots                                YES... NO...
5) I used improvised Pads                           YES... NO...
6) Having Heart Palpitations                        YES... NO...
7) Feeling Dizzy                                    YES... NO ...
8) Having Blackouts                                 YES... NO...
9) This Period came too soon from last one  YES...NO...
10) Getting Tired easily                            YES... NO...
11) I think my HB is less than 10g/dl               YES...NO...
12) I Missed my Period                              YES...NO...

If you answered YES to any of the statements above, you probably lost too much blood in this cycle. It is recommended you seek medical advice. You could also be at Risk of Ascending Infection.

i4U

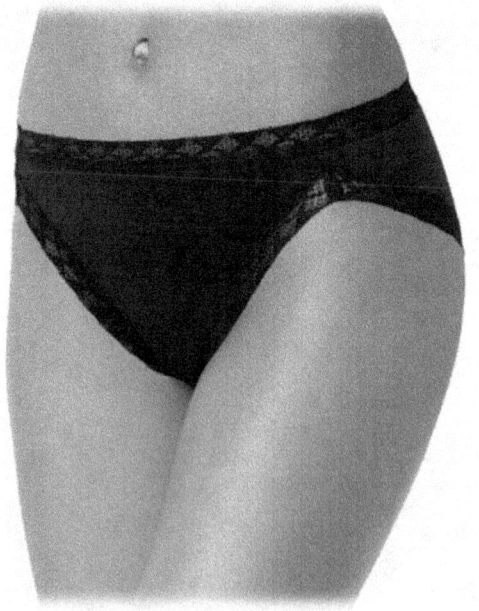

Before you go, Record the number of Pads used in this Cycle in the Table below:

| Day of Menses | # of Standard Pads used | Or Number of Tampons used | # Improvised Pads used |
|---|---|---|---|
| | SOAKED (x) | NOT SOAKED (y) | |
| Day 1 | | | |
| Day 2 | | | |
| Day 3 | | | |
| Day 4 | | | |
| Day 5 | | | |
| Day 6 | | | |
| Day 7 | | | |
| | | | |
| | Total: | Total: | |
| | | | |

Which of the Following Complaints did you experience 7 to 10 days before your period?

| | | |
|---|---|---|
| 1. | Breast PAIN | YES/ NO |
| 2. | Nausea & Vomiting | YES/NO |
| 3. | HEADACHE | YES/NO |
| 4. | DEPRESSION or Feeling Low | YES/NO |
| 5. | LOSS OF APPETITE | YES/NO |
| 6. | CONSTIPATION | YES/NO |
| 7. | BACKACHE | YES/NO |
| 8. | ANGER | YES/NO |
| 9. | IRRITABLE | YES/NO |
| 10. | AGITATION | YES/NO |
| 11. | LACK OF SELF CONTROL | YES/NO |
| 12. | Difficulties with concentration | YES/NO |
| 13. | TIREDNESS | YES/NO |
| 14. | INSOMNIA | YES/NO |

15. WRITE OTHER COMPLAINTS YOU MAY EXPERIENCE WHICH ARE NOT LISTED ABOVE

If you answered YES to most of these statements, you probably experienced pre menstrual tension or could be suffering from pre menstrual syndrome. Consult your gyneacologist for advise.

*i4U-Information for you*

# Managing Premenstrual Syndrome (PMS)

### About this information
This information is for you if you have, or think you have, premenstrual syndrome (PMS) and want to know more about it. It may also be helpful if you are a partner, relative or friend of someone who is affected by PMS.

### Key points:

**PMS is the name given to the physical and emotional symptoms affecting your daily life in the 2 weeks before you have your period.**

These symptoms usually get better once your period starts.

You should record your symptoms in this diary over two menstrual cycles in a row to help your healthcare professional make a diagnosis.

There is a wide range of options to help manage your symptoms and allow you to get on with your daily life.

Whatever option you choose, continue to keep a diary of your symptoms for at least another 2–3 months, as this can help to see whether a particular treatment is working.

### What is PMS?
PMS is the name given to the physical and emotional symptoms affecting your daily life in the 2 weeks before you have your period.

*i4U*

These symptoms usually get better once your period starts and often disappear by the end of your period.

Nearly all women have some premenstrual symptoms. Each woman's symptoms are different, but the most common include:

> - mood swings
> - feeling depressed, irritable or bad-tempered
> - feeling upset, anxious or emotional
> - tiredness or having trouble sleeping
> - headaches
> - changes in appetite and food cravings
> - feeling clumsy
> - fluid retention and feeling bloated
> - changes to skin or hair
> - sore or tender breasts.

Symptoms can vary from month to month, although they tend to form a pattern over time.

Between 2 and 4 in 100 women get PMS that is severe enough to prevent them from getting on with their daily lives. A very small number of women get an even more intense form of PMS known as premenstrual dysphoric disorder (PMDD), which is not covered in this information. If you have questions about this, you should discuss it with your healthcare professional

**What causes PMS?**

The exact cause of PMS is not known. It could be linked to changes in the levels of your hormones and body chemicals.

The levels of your hormones change during your menstrual cycle. Some women are more sensitive to these hormonal changes, which can lead to the symptoms described. Women who use some forms of hormonal contraception are less affected by PMS. PMS has also been linked to a variety of chemical substances in your blood called neurotransmitters, such as serotonin and gamma-aminobutyric acid (GABA).

**How do I know I have PMS?**
If you are getting symptoms, you should write them down in a diary for at least two menstrual cycles in a row. Your healthcare professional will then review your diary with you to see whether your symptoms fit the pattern of PMS.

If your symptom diary alone is not enough for diagnosis, you may be offered treatment with gonadotrophin-releasing hormone (GnRH) analogues for a period of 3 months. This will temporarily stop your ovaries producing hormones, which may help with your diagnosis.

**What are my options?**
There is a wide range of options to help you to manage your symptoms and allow you to get on with your daily life. Your healthcare professional will discuss these with you.

Whatever option you choose, you will be advised to continue to keep a diary of your symptoms for at least another 2–3 months, as this can help to see whether a particular treatment is working.

**Lifestyle changes**
In the first instance, you can take some positive steps to try to improve your symptoms by:

- doing more exercise

- eating a healthy balanced diet

- trying to reduce and manage stress, for example by using meditation, yoga and mindfulness.

- Speak with your healthcare professional if you would like further information about ways to change your lifestyle and about treatments that can help.

### Psychological support and therapy

Cognitive behavioural therapy (CBT) is known to help PMS symptoms and should be offered to you as a treatment option. This involves discussing your symptoms with a therapist. It can help you learn new ways of managing some of your symptoms to reduce their impact on your daily life.

### Complementary therapy

There are several alternative or complementary therapies for PMS. Many women find these helpful, although there is little evidence to show that they are effective.

You should inform your healthcare professional if you are taking any medicine or supplement. This is because some complementary therapies may react with other medicines.

Supplements of calcium, vitamin D, *Vitex agnus-castus* (a herb known as chaste berry) or *Ginkgo biloba* may be helpful. Evening primrose oil can reduce breast tenderness.

## Medical treatment
### Non-hormonal

Two types of antidepressant medications have been shown to help PMS symptoms, namely selective serotonin reuptake inhibitors (SSRIs) and serotonin–noradrenaline reuptake inhibitors (SNRIs).

Antidepressants should only be prescribed by a healthcare professional. These can be taken on a daily basis for 2 weeks before your period or all the way through your cycle.

Side effects may include nausea (feeling sick), insomnia (difficulty sleeping), tiredness and low libido (not being interested in having sex).

SSRIs are recommended as one of the first-choice treatments for severe PMS.

If you choose to stop taking antidepressants, it is important that you do so gradually so that you do not get withdrawal symptoms, such as headaches. Your healthcare team will advise you.

If you are planning a pregnancy or if you get pregnant, you should talk to your healthcare professional before stopping any medication.

Water tablets (diuretics) such as spironolactone may help some women with some physical symptoms of PMS.

**Hormonal**

## Combined oral contraceptive pill

Some women find using the combined oral contraceptive pill helps with PMS symptoms. Newer types of contraceptive pills containing a progestogen called drospirenone have been shown to improve PMS symptoms. These are considered as first-choice treatments. You may be advised to take these pills continuously, without a break, for better symptom control.

**Estrogen hormone patches or gel**

Using estrogen hormone patches or gel can improve the physical and psychological symptoms of PMS.

Unless you have had a hysterectomy (removal of your uterus), estrogen hormone patches or gel must be used in combination with a low dose of the hormone progestogen to prevent abnormal thickening of the lining of your womb. Progestogens may be given in the form of tablets (taken for a minimum of 10 days each month), pessaries or a hormone-containing coil.

Estrogen hormone patches or gel do not work as a contraceptive and so you will still need to use a method of birth control.

**Danazol**

Danazol (a synthetic hormone) in low doses can sometimes be used in the second half of your menstrual cycle to reduce breast tenderness. However, your healthcare professional should discuss with you the potential permanent side effects, such as deepening of your voice and enlargement of your clitoris.

It is important to use contraception while using danazol because it can affect the development of a female baby in the uterus.

**Gonadotrophin-releasing hormone (GnRH) analogues**

GnRH analogues may be recommended if you have severe PMS symptoms and when other treatments have not worked or are not suitable. These may also be used to help reach a diagnosis in some women, as mentioned in the *How do I know I have PMS?* section above.

These medicines cause a temporary and reversible menopause, so you will not release eggs and you will not have any periods.

If you use GnRH analogues for more than 6 months, it may affect your bone strength (osteoporosis). You will be advised to take hormone replacement therapy (HRT) to protect your bones and reduce your menopausal symptoms, such as hot flushes.

You will be advised to have regular bone density scans to check for osteoporosis if you use this treatment for more than 2 years.

You should also make sure that you get regular exercise, have a balanced diet and do not smoke.

**Surgical treatment**

Your healthcare professional will only suggest surgical treatment if you have severe symptoms and all other treatments have not helped.

Removal of your uterus along with both ovaries and fallopian tubes can help to improve severe PMS symptoms by making you menopausal.

If you have surgical treatment for PMS, you may be advised to use HRT to prevent menopausal symptoms. If your uterus and ovaries have been removed, this will be estrogen-only HRT. If you still have your uterus, you will need both estrogen and progestogen. Progestogens protect the lining of your uterus, but may then re-introduce symptoms of PMS.

If you are considering surgical treatment, your healthcare professional will advise you to use GnRH analogues and HRT for 3–6 months before surgery. GnRH analogues have a similar effect on your hormones as having your ovaries removed and will give you an idea of how you may feel after the operation. You may also be able to see whether you will benefit from surgery and whether HRT suits you.

Surgical treatment such as endometrial ablation or hysterectomy without removal of both ovaries is not recommended for treatment of PMS.

**At what stage of treatment should I be referred to a gynaecologist?**

If simple measures such as combined pills or SSRIs have not worked, your GP will refer you to a specialist. A team of healthcare professionals may be involved in your care, including your GP, a nurse specialist, a dietician, a mental health professional (psychiatrist, clinical psychologist or counsellor) and a gynaecologist. The make-up of the team will depend on the hospital you attend.

**Reproduced from: Royal College of Obstetricians and Gynaecologists. Managing Premenstrual Syndrome patient information leaflet, London,**

i4U

RCOG, Mar 2018, with the permission of the
Royal College of Obstetricians and Gynaecologists.

February 20......

happy valentines

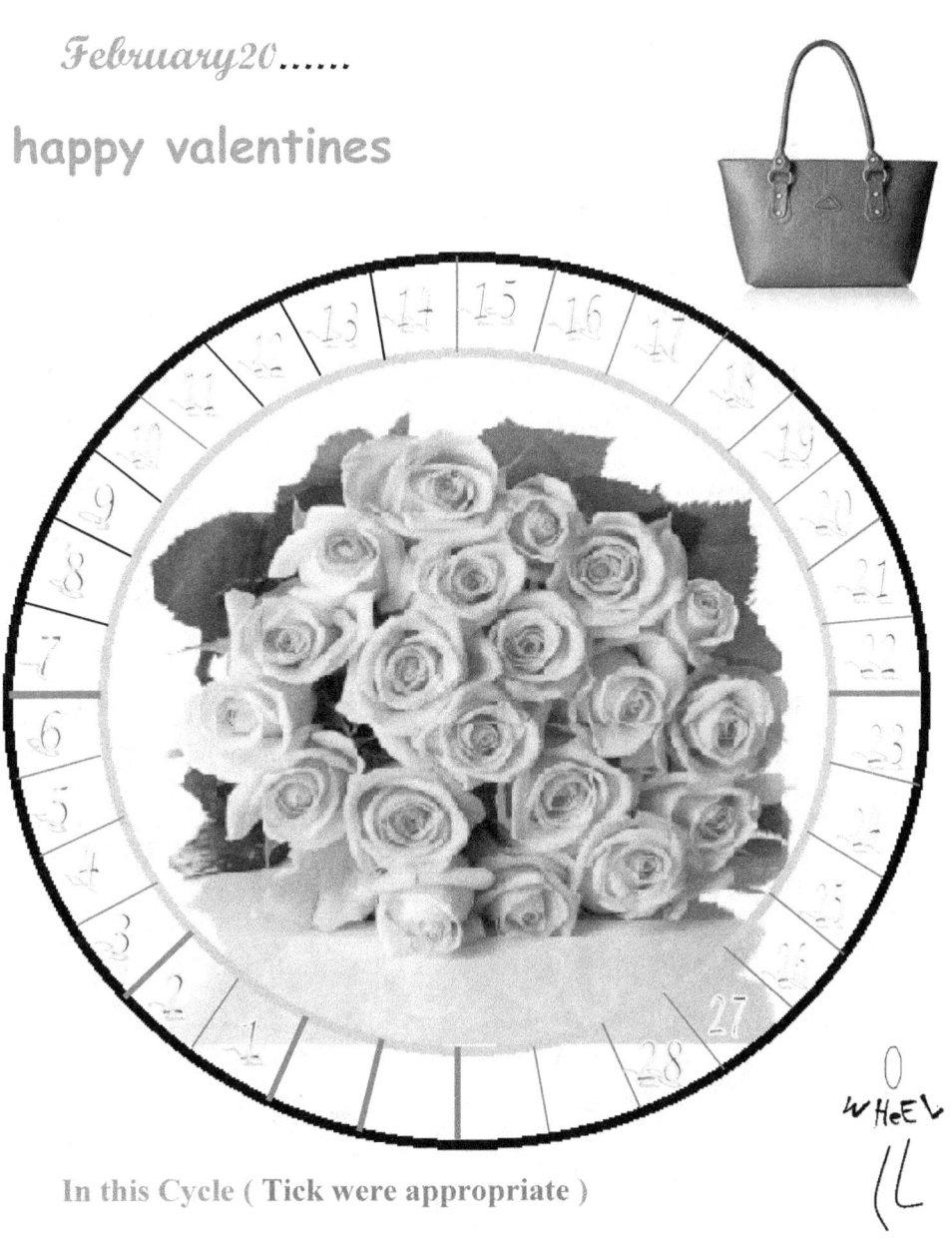

In this Cycle ( Tick were appropriate )

WHEEL

i4U

1) Period lasted longer than seven days     YES... NO...
2) Used more pads than is usual for me     YES...NO...
3) Feeling ill     YES...NO...
4) I used Improvised pads     YES... NO...
5) More pads soaked than is usual for me     YES... NO...
6) Tampons soaked than is usual for me     YES... NO...
7) I had painful menses     YES... NO...
8) Heart beating too Fast     YES... NO...
9) Having Heart Palpitations     YES... NO...
10) Feeling Dizzy     YES... NO ...
11) Having Blackouts     YES... NO...
12) This Period came too soon from last one     YES...NO...
13) Getting Tired easily     YES...NO...
14) I think my HB is less than 10g/dl     YES...NO...
15) I Missed my Period     YES...NO...
16) WRITE OTHER COMPLAINTS YOU MAY EXPERIENCE THAT ARE NOT LISTED ABOVE

If you answered YES to any of the statements above, you probably lost too much blood in this cycle. It is recommended you seek medical advice.

**Before you go, Record the number of Pads or Tampons used in this Cycle in the Table below:**

| Day of Menses | # of Standard Pads used | Or Number of Tampons used | # Improvised Pads used |
|---|---|---|---|
| | SOAKED (x) | NOT SOAKED (y) | |
| Day 1 | | | |
| Day 2 | | | |
| Day 3 | | | |
| Day 4 | | | |
| Day 5 | | | |
| Day 6 | | | |
| Day 7 | | | |
| | | | |
| | Total: | Total : | |
| | | | |

Which of the Following Complaints did you experience 7 to 10 days before your period

*i4U*

1) Severe Abdominal PAIN        YES/ NO
2) Vomiting                     YES/NO

| | | |
|---|---|---|
| 3) | NAUSEA | YES/NO |
| 4) | HEADACHE | YES/NO |
| 5) | DEPRESSION or Feeling Low | YES/NO |
| 6) | LOSS OF APPETITE | YES/NO |
| 7) | CONSTIPATION | YES/NO |
| 8) | BACKACHE | YES/NO |
| 9) | ANGER | YES/NO |
| 10) | IRRITABLE | YES/NO |
| 11) | AGITATION | YES/NO |
| 12) | LACK OF SELF CONTROL | YES/NO |
| 13) | Difficulties with concentration | YES/NO |
| 14) | TIREDNESS | YES/NO |
| 15) | INSOMNIA | YES/NO |

If you answered YES to most of these statements, you probably experienced pre Menstrual tension or could be suffering from pre menstrual syndrome. Consult your gyneacologist for advice.

1. COST OF SANITARY PADS/TAMPONS USED THIS MONTH: ......

2. BUDGET FOR PADS/TAMPONS NEXT MONTH: ......

i4U

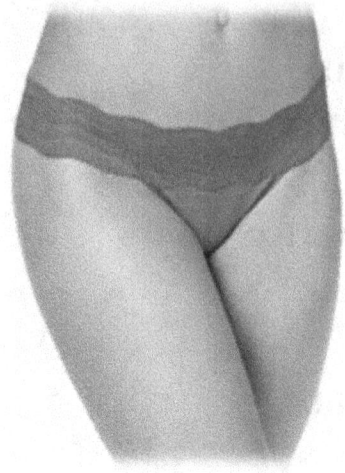

*i4U – Information for you*

## Chronic (long-term) pelvic pain

### About this information

This information is for you if you want to know more about chronic pelvic pain. It may also be helpful if you are a relative or friend of someone who has chronic pelvic pain.

### What is chronic pelvic pain?

Pelvic pain is pain that you feel in your lower abdomen or pelvis. Pain is described as 'chronic' if it occurs all or some of the time for more than 6 months. Chronic pelvic pain is a description of the symptoms you are experiencing.

It is common and affects around 1 in 6 women. It can be distressing and affect quality of life and a woman's ability to carry out everyday activities.

### What causes chronic pelvic pain?

Chronic pelvic pain is usually caused by a combination of physical, psychological and/or social factors rather than a single underlying condition, although for many women a cause cannot be found.

Possible causes include:

- endometriosis, a condition where the cells of the lining of the womb (endometrium) are found elsewhere in the body, usually in the pelvis – endometriosis and adenomyosis (a condition where the endometrium is found in the muscle of the womb) can cause pain around the time of a period and during sex
- pelvic inflammatory disease, which is an infection in the fallopian tubes and/or pelvis
- interstitial cystitis (bladder inflammation)
- adhesions (areas of scarred tissue that may be a result of a previous infection, endometriosis or surgery)
- trapped or damaged nerves in the pelvic area

> pelvic organ prolapse
> musculoskeletal pain (pain in the joints, muscles, ligaments and bones of the pelvis)
> irritable bowel syndrome (IBS)
> depression, including postnatal depression
> traumatic experiences, such as sexual and/or physical abuse.

Your doctor will be able to rule out any serious problems that you may be worried about.

**What will happen when I see the doctor?**

At your appointment, you should have the opportunity to describe the pain you are having and to discuss your concerns.

The way you describe your symptoms is important in making a diagnosis. You should tell your doctor about:

> the pattern of your pain
> what makes your pain better or worse (certain kinds of movement or position, for example)
> what medication you have tried
> whether you have noticed other problems that might be linked to the pain, for example with your periods, sex, bladder or bowel, or psychological symptoms.

You may be asked to keep a pain diary where you note down when your pain occurs, how severe it is, how long it lasts and what seems to affect it, for example your periods.

You may be asked about aspects of your everyday life including your sleep patterns, appetite and general wellbeing. You may be asked whether you currently or in the past have experienced physical or sexual abuse.

You may also be asked whether you are feeling depressed or tearful. This is because long-term pain is known to cause depression, which in turn may make your pain worse. Knowing how your pain affects you means this can be taken into account in deciding on the most appropriate treatment for you.

If you have bladder, bowel or psychological symptoms, you may be referred to other specialists as part of your investigations and the treatment offered.

After you have described your symptoms you may be offered:

➢ an examination of your abdomen
➢ a vaginal examination.

Your doctor will listen to you and take your concerns seriously. By working in partnership with you, he or she will aim to identify the possible cause of your pain and offer the most appropriate treatment.

**What tests might I be offered?**

➢ screening tests for pelvic infections (including sexually transmitted infections)
➢ an ultrasound scan – this may be a trans-vaginal scan of your pelvis, which involves gently inserting an ultrasound probe into your vagina
➢ an MRI (magnetic resonance imaging) scan of your pelvis.

You may also be offered a laparoscopy, particularly if your doctor thinks you may have endometriosis, adhesions or pelvic infection. This is an operation carried out under general anaesthetic. It usually involves two or three small cuts in the abdomen. A narrow telescope (called a laparoscope) is inserted through the abdominal wall to examine your pelvis. As with any surgical procedure, there are risks and benefits and these will be explained to you.

In a third to a half of laparoscopies done to investigate chronic pelvic pain, no obvious cause is found. This may be reassuring, but can also be frustrating. However, having more information can help you and your doctor decide what is the best treatment for you.

**What treatment may help?**

If your doctor thinks that your pain is due to a particular cause then you should be offered treatment for that condition:

> - irritable bowel syndrome (IBS) – medication and changes to your diet may help
>
> - infections should be treated (usually with antibiotics)
>
> - if your pain is related to your periods, you may be offered hormone treatment, for example the pill, injections or the Mirena IUS (hormone coil) to stop your periods for 3–6 months, instead of having a laparoscopy – these treatments may also be worth trying even if there is no pattern to your pain
>
> - surgery for mild adhesions does not appear to help pelvic pain – however, it may be considered in cases of severe adhesions caused by endometriosis or previous surgery.

Many women find that they can cope better with the pain if they have been listened to, taken seriously, have a full explanation of their test results and agree a plan of action. You may be reassured by finding that nothing is seriously wrong and the pain may get better with time.

Some women find acupuncture or complementary therapies, or changing diet, helpful.

Whatever your situation, you should be offered pain relief. If this does not help, you may be referred to a pain management team or a specialist pain clinic.

Chronic pelvic pain can be very difficult to live with and can cause emotional, social and economic difficulties. You may experience depression, difficulty sleeping and disruption to your daily routine. Talk to your GP if this is the case. The support of other women who also experience pelvic pain may also help: see below for information about support groups.

**Key points**

- Chronic pelvic pain is any pain in the lower abdomen or pelvis that lasts for more than 6 months.

- It is common, affecting around 1 in 6 women.

- In a third to a half of laparoscopies done to investigate chronic pelvic pain, no obvious cause is found.

- It can be due to physical, psychological and/or social factors.

- Your doctors will discuss a treatment and management plan with you.

**Reproduced from: Royal College of Obstetricians and Gynaecologists. Managing Chronic pelvic pain patient information leaflet, London, RCOG, Jul 2015, with the permission of the Royal College of Obstetricians and Gynaecologists**

i4U

*March* 20......

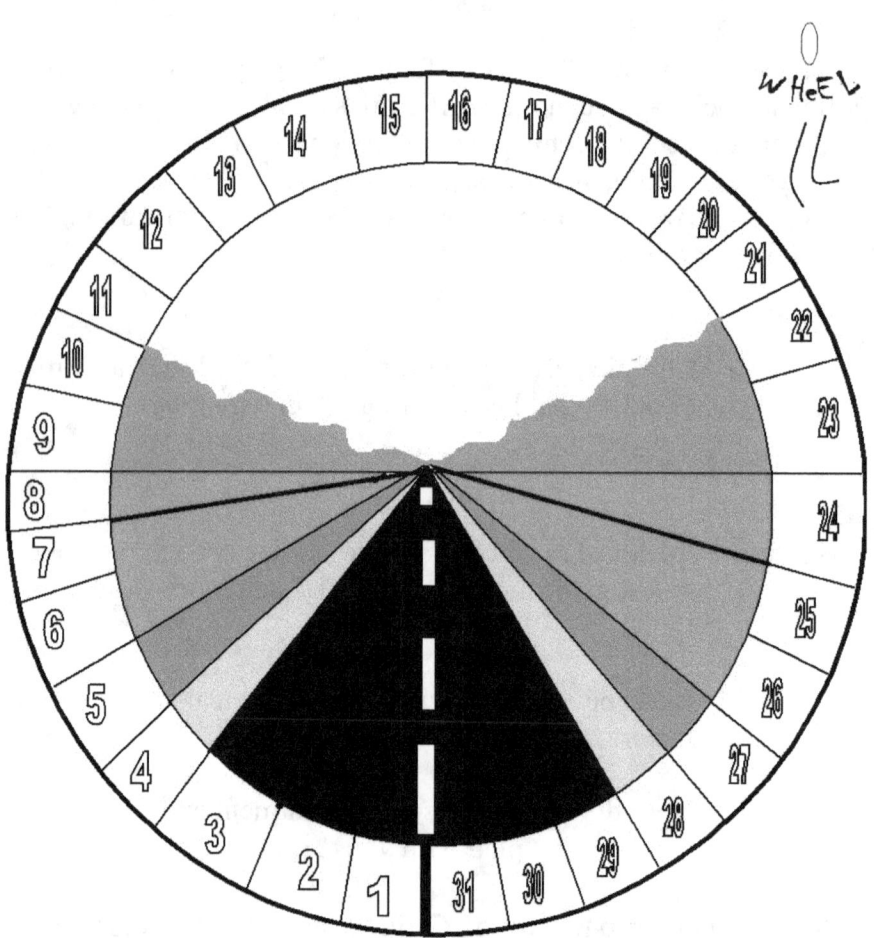

WHeEL
IL

In this Cycle ( Tick were appropriate )

1) Period lasted longer than seven days     YES... NO...
2) Used more pads than is usual for me      YES... NO...
3) Used more tampons than is usual for me   YES...NO...
4) I Bled with Clots                        YES... NO...

5) More pads soaked than is usual for me   YES... NO...
6) Tampons soaked than is usual for me    YES...NO...
7) I used improvised Pads                  YES... NO...
8) Heart beating too Fast                  YES... NO...
9) Having Heart Palpitations               YES... NO...
10) Feeling Dizzy                          YES... NO...
11) Having Blackouts                       YES... NO...
12) Period came too soon from last one     YES...NO...
13) Getting Tired easily                   YES...NO...
14) I think my HB is less than 8g/dl       YES...NO...
15) I Missed my Period                     YES...NO...
16) **WRITE OTHER COMPLAINTS YOU MAY EXPERIENCE WHICH ARE NOT LISTED ABOVE**

If you answered YES to any of the statements above, you probably lost too much blood in this cycle. It is recommended you seek medical advice.

Before you go, Record the number of Pads used in this Cycle in the Table below:

| Day of Menses | # of Standard Pads used | | Or Number of Tampons used | # Improvised Pads used |
|---|---|---|---|---|
| | SOAKED (x) | NOT SOAKED (y) | | |
| Day 1 | | | | |
| Day 2 | | | | |
| Day 3 | | | | |
| Day 4 | | | | |
| Day 5 | | | | |
| Day 6 | | | | |
| Day 7 | | | | |
| | | | | |
| | Total: | Total: | | |
| | | | | |

Which of the Following Complaints did you experience 7 to 10 days before your period?

| | |
|---|---|
| 1) Breast PAIN | YES/ NO |
| 2) Vomiting | YES/NO |
| 3) NAUSEA | YES/NO |
| 4) HEADACHE | YES/NO |
| 5) DEPRESSION or Feeling Low | YES/NO |
| 6) LOSS OF APPETITE | YES/NO |
| 7) CONSTIPATION | YES/NO |
| 8) BACKACHE | YES/NO |
| 9) ANGER | YES/NO |
| 10) IRRITABLE | YES/NO |
| 11) AGITATION | YES/NO |
| 12) LACK OF SELF CONTROL | YES/NO |
| 13) DIFFICULTIES with concentration | YES/NO |
| 14) TIREDNESS | YES/NO |
| 15) INSOMNIA | YES/NO |
| 16) I FEEL LUMPS IN MY BREASTS | YES/NO |

17) WRITE OTHER COMPLAINTS YOU MAY EXPERIENCE WHICH ARE NOT LISTED ABOVE

If you answered YES to most of these statements, you probably experienced pre Menstrual tension or could be suffering from pre menstrual syndrome. Consult your gyneacologist for advice. See a Surgeon or Nurse for advice when you feel Lumps in Your Breast.

*i4U*

# *i4U- Information for you*

# Early miscarriage

## About this information

This information is for you if you want to know more about miscarriage in the first 3 months of pregnancy. It may also be helpful if you are a relative or friend of someone who has had an early miscarriage.

This leaflet explains the care you will receive after an early miscarriage has been confirmed.

## What is an early miscarriage?

If you lose your baby in the first 3 months of pregnancy, it is called an early miscarriage. Most women experience vaginal bleeding but occasionally there may be no symptoms. If this is the case, the miscarriage may be diagnosed by an ultrasound scan.

## Why do early miscarriages happen?

In most cases, it is not possible to give a reason for an early miscarriage. The most common cause is thought to be a problem with the baby's chromosomes (the genetic structures within the body's cells that we inherit from our parents). If a baby does not have the right number of chromosomes, it will not develop properly and the pregnancy can end in a miscarriage.

## What are my chances of having a miscarriage?

Sadly, early miscarriages are very common. Many early miscarriages occur before a woman has missed her first period or before her pregnancy has been confirmed. In the first 3 months, one in five women will have a miscarriage, for no apparent reason, following a positive pregnancy test.

The risk of miscarriage is increased by:

> - your age – at the age of 30, the risk of miscarriage is one in five (20%); over the age of 40, the risk of miscarriage is one in two (50%)
> - medical problems such as poorly controlled diabetes
> - lifestyle factors such as smoking, being overweight or heavy drinking.

There is no evidence that stress can cause a miscarriage. Sex during pregnancy is not associated with early miscarriage.

## What should I do if I have bleeding and/or pain in the first 3 months?

Vaginal bleeding and/or cramping pain in the early stages of pregnancy are common and do not always mean that there is a problem. However, bleeding and/or pain can be a sign of a miscarriage.

If you have any bleeding and/or pain, you can get medical help and advice from:

> - your GP or midwife
> - your nearest Early Pregnancy Assessment Service
> - the A&E department at your local hospital, particularly if you are bleeding heavily, have severe pain or feel very unwell.

## How is an early miscarriage diagnosed?

An early miscarriage is usually diagnosed by an ultrasound scan. You may be advised to have either a trans-vaginal scan (where a probe is gently inserted in your vagina) or a trans-abdominal scan (where the probe is placed on your abdomen) or occasionally both. A trans-vaginal scan may be recommended as it gives a clearer image. Neither scan increases your risk of having a miscarriage.

You may be offered blood tests that could include checking the level of your pregnancy hormone ($\beta hCG$).

If you are bleeding or have pain, a vaginal examination may be carried out. You should be offered a chaperone (someone to accompany you) for a vaginal examination or a trans-vaginal scan. You may also wish to bring someone to support you during your examination or scan.

Some women will miscarry quite quickly but for others the diagnosis and ongoing management may take several weeks.

## What are my choices if a miscarriage is confirmed?

If your ultrasound scan shows that you have miscarried and nothing remains in your womb, you may not need any further treatment.

If the miscarriage is confirmed but some or all of the pregnancy is still inside your womb, your healthcare professional will talk to you about the best options for you. You may choose to wait and let nature take its course, or to use medicines or to have an operation.

**Letting nature take its course (expectant management of a miscarriage)**

This is successful in about 50 out of 100 women who choose this option. It can take some time before the bleeding starts and this may continue for up to 3 weeks. It may be heavy and you may experience cramping pain. If you have severe pain or very heavy bleeding, you may need to be admitted to hospital.

You should be given a follow-up appointment about 2 weeks later:

> If the bleeding and pain has settled by then, it is likely that all the pregnancy has come away. You will be advised to do a urine pregnancy test 1 week after this. If it is still positive, you should contact your local Early Pregnancy Assessment Service.

> If bleeding fails to start within 7–14 days or is persisting or getting heavier, you will be offered a further ultrasound scan. The options of continuing expectant management, medical treatment or having an operation will then be discussed with you.

**Taking medication (medical management of a miscarriage)**

This is successful in 85 out of 100 women and avoids an anaesthetic.

You will be given medication called misoprostol, usually as vaginal pessaries although tablets to swallow may be taken if you prefer. The medication helps the neck of the womb (cervix) to open and lets the remaining pregnancy come away. It will take a few hours and there will be some pain with bleeding or clotting (like a heavy period). You will be offered pain relief and anti-sickness medication. Some women may experience diarrhoea and vomiting.

If bleeding has not started 24 hours after treatment, you should contact your Early Pregnancy Assessment Service or hospital.

*i4U*

After the treatment, you may bleed for up to 3 weeks. If the bleeding is heavy, you should contact your local hospital.

You will be advised to do a pregnancy test 3 weeks later. If this is positive, you should contact your Early Pregnancy Assessment Service to arrange a follow-up appointment. If the treatment has not worked, you will be given the option of having an operation.

**Having an operation (surgical management of a miscarriage)**

The operation may be carried out under general or local anaesthetic. It is successful in 95 out of 100 women.

The pregnancy is removed through the cervix. You may be given tablets to swallow or vaginal pessaries before the operation to soften your cervix.

Surgery will usually take place within a few days of your miscarriage but you may be advised to have surgery immediately if:

- you are bleeding heavily and continuously
- there are signs of infection
- medical treatment to remove the pregnancy has been unsuccessful.

The operation is safe but there is a small risk of complications including heavy bleeding, infection or damage to the womb. A repeat operation is sometimes required. The risk of infection is the same if you choose medical or surgical treatment.

**What happens to the pregnancy remains?**

Some tissue removed at the time of surgery may be sent for testing in the laboratory. The results can confirm that the pregnancy was inside the womb and not an ectopic pregnancy (when the pregnancy is growing outside the womb). It also tests for any abnormal changes in the placenta (molar pregnancy).

Some women who miscarry at home choose to bring pregnancy remains to the hospital so that they can be tested.

Options for disposal of the remains will be discussed with you and your partner.

**I would like to have a memorial for my baby. How do I organise that?**

Depending on your unit and your own individual circumstances, you may choose burial or cremation. Many hospitals have a book of remembrance. If you would like further information, talk to your doctor or nurse about the options at your hospital.

**What happens next?**

**Vaginal bleeding**

You can expect to have some vaginal bleeding for 1–2 weeks after your miscarriage. This is like a heavy period for the first day or so. This should lessen and may become brown in colour. You should use sanitary towels rather than tampons, as using tampons could increase the risk of infection.

If you normally have regular periods, your next period will usually be in 4–6 weeks' time. Ovulation occurs before this, so you may be fertile in the first month after a miscarriage. Therefore, if you do not want to become pregnant, you will need to use contraception.

**Discomfort**

You can expect some cramps (like strong period pains) in your lower abdomen on the day of your miscarriage. You may get milder cramps or an ache for a day or so afterwards. If the discomfort is not relieved by simple painkillers from the pharmacy and you experience the following symptoms, you should seek medical advice from your GP, Early Pregnancy Assessment Service or the hospital where you had your care.

**Heavy or prolonged vaginal bleeding, smelly vaginal discharge and abdominal pain:** If you also have a raised temperature (fever) and flu-like symptoms, you may have an infection of the lining of the womb (uterus). This occurs in two to three out of 100 women. It can be treated with antibiotics. These symptoms can also indicate that some tissue remains from the pregnancy (see above).

**Increasing abdominal pain and you feel unwell:** If you also have a temperature (fever), have lost your appetite and are vomiting, this may be due to damage to your uterus. You may need to be admitted to hospital.

## Emotional recovery

A miscarriage affects every woman differently and can be devastating for her partner too. Some women come to terms with what has happened within weeks; for others, it takes longer. Many women feel tearful and emotional for a short time afterwards. Some women experience intense grief over a longer time.

Your family and friends may be able to help. Talk to your GP if you feel you are not coping.

**Returning to work**

When you return to work depends on you and how you feel. It is advisable to rest for a few days before starting your routine activities but returning to work within a day or two will not cause you harm if you feel well enough. Most women will return to work in a week, but you may need longer to recover emotionally. If so, it may be helpful to talk with your GP or occupational health adviser.

**Having sex**

You can have sex as soon as you both feel ready. It is important that you are feeling well and that any pain and bleeding has significantly reduced.

**When can we try for another baby?**

You can try for a baby as soon as you and your partner feel physically and emotionally ready.

**Am I at higher risk of a miscarriage next time?**

You are not at higher risk of another miscarriage if you have had one or two early miscarriages. Most miscarriages occur as a one-off event and there is a good chance of having a successful pregnancy in the future.

A very small number of women have a condition that makes them more likely to miscarry. If this is the case, medication may help.

**Is there anything else I should know?**

Like anyone else planning to have a baby, you should:

> - take 400 micrograms of folic acid every day from when you start trying until 12 weeks of pregnancy to reduce the risk of your baby being born with a neural tube defect (spina bifida)
> - be as healthy as you can – eat a balanced diet and stop smoking

➢ not drink alcohol as this may increase your chance of miscarriage

**Key points**

Early miscarriages are very common and one in five women have a miscarriage for no apparent reason.

Bleeding and/or pain in early pregnancy can be a warning sign of miscarriage and you should seek medical advice if you are in this situation.

You may be offered tests including an ultrasound scan to check your pregnancy.

Once a miscarriage is diagnosed, your healthcare professional will tell you about your options, which include expectant, medical or surgical treatment.

Most miscarriages are a one-off event and there is a good chance of a successful pregnancy in future.

**Reproduced from: Royal College of Obstetricians and Gynaecologists. Early Miscarriage patient information leaflet, London, RCOG, Sept 2016, with the permission of the Royal College of Obstetricians and Gynaecologists**

*April* 20......

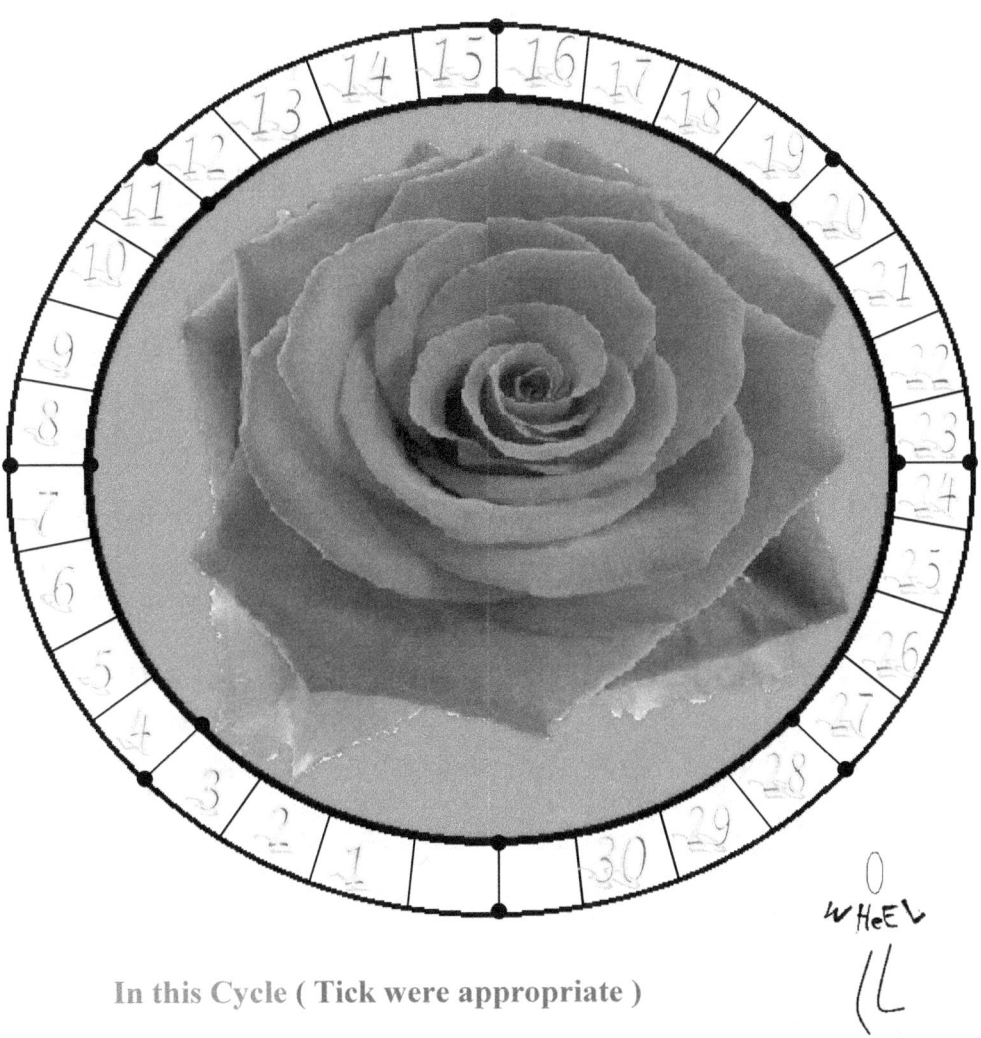

In this Cycle ( Tick were appropriate )

1) Period lasted longer than seven days    YES... NO...
2) Used more pads than is usual for me    YES... NO...
3) Used more tampons than usual    YES...NO...
4) I Bled with Clots    YES... NO...

i4U

| | |
|---|---|
| 5) More pads soaked than usual | YES… NO… |
| 6) More tampons soaked than usual | YES… NO… |
| 7) I Fainted | YES… NO… |
| 8) Heart beating too Fast | YES… NO… |
| 9) Having Heart Palpitations | YES… NO… |
| 10) Feeling Dizzy | YES… NO … |
| 11) Having Blackouts | YES… NO… |
| 12) This Period came too soon | YES…. NO… |
| 13) Getting Tired easily | YES…NO… |
| 14) I think my HB is less than 7g/dl | YES…NO… |
| 15) I Missed my Period | YES…NO… |

**16) WRITE OTHER COMPLAINTS YOU MAY EXPERIENCE WHICH ARE NOT LISTED ABOVE**

If you answered YES to any of the statements above, you probably lost too much blood in this cycle. It is recommended you see your Doctor for a check up.

Before you go, Record the number of Pads or Tampons used in this Cycle in the Table below:

| Day of Menses | # of Standard Pads used | Or Number of Tampons used | # Improvised Pads used |
|---|---|---|---|
| | SOAKED | NOT SOAKED | |

|  | (x) | (y) |  |
|---|---|---|---|
| Day 1 |  |  |  |
| Day 2 |  |  |  |
| Day 3 |  |  |  |
| Day 4 |  |  |  |
| Day 5 |  |  |  |
| Day 6 |  |  |  |
| Day 7 |  |  |  |
|  |  |  |  |
|  | Total: | Total : |  |
|  |  |  |  |

**Which of the Following Complaints did you experience 7 to 10 days before your period?**

1) Breast PAIN           YES/ NO
2) Vomiting              YES/NO

3) NAUSEA  YES/NO
4) HEADACHE  YES/NO
5) DEPRESSION or Feeling Low  YES/NO
6) LOSS OF APPETITE  YES/NO
7) CONSTIPATION  YES/NO
8) BACKACHE  YES/NO
9) ANGER  YES/NO
10) IRRITABLE  YES/NO
11) AGITATION  YES/NO
12) LACK OF SELF CONTROL  YES/NO
13) DIFFICULTIES with concentration  YES/NO
14) TIREDNESS  YES/NO
15) INSOMNIA  YES/NO
16) I Feel Lumps in my Breasts  YES/NO
17) WRITE OTHER COMPLAINTS YOU MAY EXPERIENCE WHICH ARE NOT LISTED ABOVE

If you answered YES to most of these statements, you probably experienced pre Menstrual tension or could be suffering from pre menstrual syndrome. Consult your gyneacologist for advice. See a Surgeon or Nurse for advice on Lumps in Your Breast.

# i4U – Information for You

# Choosing to have a caesarean section

## About this information

This information is for you if you are thinking about having your baby by a 'planned' or 'elective' caesarean section when there isn't a 'medical' reason to do so. If you are a partner or relative of someone in this situation, you may also find it helpful.

This information is *not* for you if you have a complicated pregnancy, because the balance of benefits and risks will be different. If you are in that situation, your obstetrician and midwife will talk with you about your options for birth.

## Why isn't caesarean section recommended for every woman?

Most women in the UK give birth vaginally, recover well and have healthy babies.

Most women who have a planned caesarean section will also recover well and have healthy babies. However, there are risks for both you and your baby and it may take longer to get back to normal after your baby is born. Having a caesarean section also makes future births more complicated.

Doctors will not recommend a caesarean section unless it is necessary for medical reasons.

## I am thinking about having a caesarean section. Who should I speak to?

Talk to your midwife about why you would like a caesarean section. You may also wish to talk to other members of your healthcare team, such as your obstetrician or an anaesthetist.

It is important that you tell your midwife as early as possible in your pregnancy. This is so that there is time to talk about your concerns

i4U

and wishes and to arrange appointments with other health professionals who may be able to help.

Feel free to be honest about your feelings and concerns so that your midwife and obstetrician can give you the support you need to make a decision.

**Reasons why you may be thinking about having a caesarean section**

It is important that you explore the reasons why you are thinking of a caesarean section. There may be other options to consider, such as in the examples below:

- You may have had a complicated vaginal birth in the past. Talk to your midwife and obstetrician about your birth experience. They can explain that not all labours are the same. Going through your notes with someone and talking through what happened last time can help you make up your mind.
- You may believe that it is safer to have a caesarean section or have concerns that vaginal birth is more likely to damage your pelvic floor. You can find more information about the risks involved below.
- You may have anxieties about having a vaginal birth for the first time. Often talking through what happens during labour and birth, your choices for pain relief and hearing what support you will have may be enough to reassure you to think about a vaginal birth.
- You may have concerns about when you are likely to have your baby. For example, if your partner works away from home for long periods, you may think your only option is a caesarean section. In this situation you could consider having your labour started (which is known as being induced) instead. If you choose this option, your doctor or midwife will talk to you about the implications for you and your baby.
- You may have a fear of having a vaginal birth (tokophobia) or vaginal examinations. You may have had a previous traumatic experience such as rape or child

abuse. You should have the opportunity to talk to a specialist who will help you manage your anxiety and therefore increase your ability to cope if you wish to try for a vaginal birth. These skills can be used to help you feel more in control.

Your obstetrician or midwife will explain the risks and benefits of caesarean section compared with a vaginal birth. They will ensure that you have the right support to help you choose the right birth for you and your family.

**What will a caesarean section mean for me and my baby?**

It is important that you consider the risks and benefits carefully. People view risk differently and how you view risk depends to a large extent on your own circumstances and experience.

**For you**

Having a planned caesarean section may make you feel more in control and avoid the anxieties and uncertainties of going into labour naturally. However, it is surgery and can have complications. It will also affect your future pregnancies (see below).

Although you should not feel any pain during the caesarean section (because you will have an anaesthetic), the wound will be sore for the first few days. One in 10 women will experience discomfort for the first few months.

The main risks when having a caesarean section include:

> ➢ wound infection – this is common and can take several weeks to heal

> blood clots in the legs that can travel to the lungs (deep vein thrombosis and pulmonary embolism) – these are more common with a caesarean.
> bleeding more than expected.

These risks are increased if you are overweight.

Serious complications are rare if it is your first caesarean section and it is planned in advance, as long as you are fit and healthy and are not overweight. However, serious complications become more common if you have repeated caesarean sections. See the section below on future births.

If you develop any complications, your recovery and stay in hospital will be longer.

**For your baby**

The most common problem affecting babies born by caesarean section is temporary breathing difficulty. Your baby is more likely to need care on the neonatal unit than a baby born vaginally.

There is a small risk of your baby being cut during the operation. This is usually a small cut that isn't deep. This happens in 1 to 2 out of every 100 babies delivered by caesarean section, but usually heals without any further harm. Thin adhesive strips may be needed to seal the wound while it heals.

Babies born by caesarean section are more likely to develop asthma in childhood and to become overweight.

**What about the effect on future births?**

If you choose to have a caesarean section, any future births are more likely to be by caesarean section as well. You should consider the size of the family you want because the risks increase with the number of caesarean sections you have. Two caesarean sections do not appear to have a higher complication rate, but three or more carry serious risks which include the following:

- Damage to your bowel or bladder (1 in 1000 women) or ureter (the tube connecting the kidney to the bladder) (3 in 10 000 women).
- Extra procedures that may become necessary during the caesarean section such as a blood transfusion or emergency hysterectomy, particularly if there is heavy bleeding at the time of your caesarean section. A hysterectomy would mean you are unable to have any further children. The risk of needing to undergo a hysterectomy at the end of a subsequent pregnancy increases with each caesarean section but overall is still very low.
- If you have had two caesarean sections before and have a low placenta in your third pregnancy, you have a higher chance of a serious complication called placenta accreta. This is where the placenta does not come away as it should when your baby is delivered. If this is the case, you may lose a lot of blood and need a blood transfusion, and you are likely to need a hysterectomy. The risk of placenta accreta increases with each caesarean section.
- For reasons we don't yet understand, the chances of experiencing a stillbirth in a future pregnancy are higher if you have had a caesarean section (4 in 1000 women) compared with a vaginal birth (2 in 1000 women).

## How does a vaginal birth compare?

Having a vaginal birth is usually straightforward, particularly if you have had a vaginal birth before. It is normal for the area between your vagina and anus (perineum) to feel sore and uncomfortable for a while after you have given birth. This is because this area will have stretched as your baby is born and you may have stitches.

Complications can also happen, especially with first births. These include the need for forceps or ventouse to help deliver your baby. Heavy bleeding in the first few days is more likely with a vaginal birth than with a caesarean section. However, there is generally more blood lost with a caesarean section overall.

## What are the benefits of having a vaginal birth?

If you do have a vaginal birth, it is worth remembering that:

> you are more likely to be able to have skin-to-skin contact with your baby immediately after birth and to be able to breastfeed successfully your recovery is likely to be quicker, you should be able to get back to everyday activities more quickly and you should be able to drive sooner if you have had a vaginal birth with your first baby, future labours are usually much shorter and the risks are very low to you and your baby.

## I've thought about it carefully and I still want a caesarean section

If you are certain that you do not want a vaginal birth and understand the risks of a caesarean section and the impact on future births, you can ask for a caesarean section. If your obstetrician does not feel that he or she can support your decision to have a caesarean section, you can ask to be referred to another consultant to discuss this. There are maternity units that do not offer caesarean section on request and therefore you may be referred to a different maternity unit.

## If I choose a caesarean section, when will it be done?

You will usually be offered a date after 39 weeks of pregnancy. Babies born by caesarean section earlier than this are more likely to need to be admitted to the neonatal unit for help with their breathing.

The planned date might have to be changed, if someone else's need is more urgent. If this is the case, the doctors and midwives will arrange a new date with you.

## What anaesthetic will I have?

There are two types of anaesthetic. You can be either awake (a regional anaesthetic) or asleep (a general anaesthetic). The majority of women having a planned caesarean section will have a regional anaesthetic (a spinal anaesthetic or an epidural, or a combination of the two). This is where you are awake and will not feel pain although you may feel pulling or pressure in your lower body. It is usually safer for you and your baby than a general anaesthetic and allows you and your partner to experience the birth together.

You will have an opportunity to discuss your anaesthetic with an anaesthetist. For more information on the different types of anaesthetic and risks of each, see www.labourpains.com, which is the public information website of the Obstetric Anaesthetists' Association.

**Can I still have a caesarean section if I go into labour before the planned date for my operation?**

One in 10 women go into labour before the date of their planned caesarean section. If there is no 'medical' need for a caesarean section, you are likely to be offered the chance to continue in labour and aim for a vaginal birth, particularly if labour is advanced. Your midwife and doctor will discuss this with you at the time.

If you still decide to have the caesarean section as planned, it will be performed as soon as possible.

**Key points**

Most women in the UK give birth vaginally, recover well and have healthy babies.

Although there are risks with a vaginal birth, if you have had a vaginal birth with your first baby, future labours are usually much shorter and the risks are very low for you and your baby.

Most women who have a planned caesarean section will also recover well and have healthy babies but there are risks for both you and your baby and it takes longer to get back to normal after your baby is born.

Having a caesarean section may make future births more complicated.

**Reproduced from: Royal College of Obstetricians and Gynaecologists. Choosing to have a caesarean section patient information leaflet, London, RCOG, Jul 2015, with the permission of the Royal College of Obstetricians and Gynaecologists**

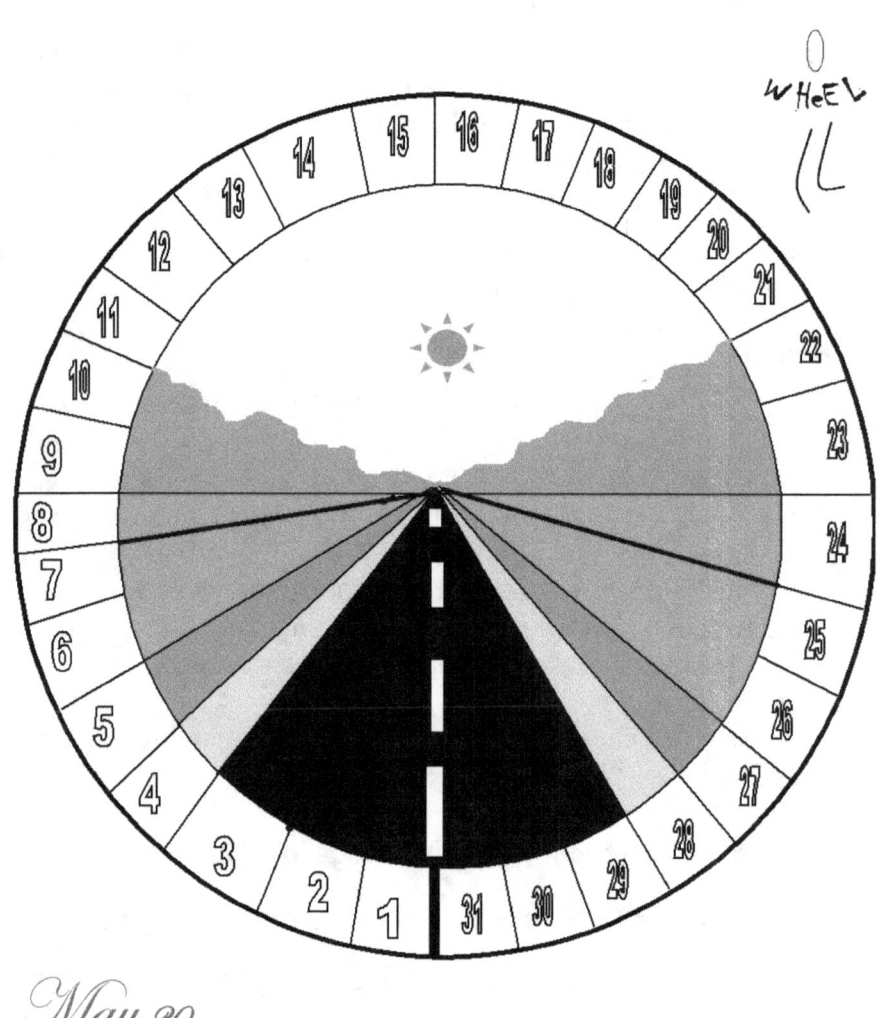

May 20......

**In this Cycle ( Tick were appropriate )**

    1) **Period lasted longer than seven days**    YES… NO...

    2) **Used more pads than usual**    YES… NO…

3) Used more tampons than usual for          YES… NO…
4) I Bled with Clots                         YES… NO…
5) More pads soaked than is usual for me     YES… NO…
6) More tampons soaked than usual            YES… NO…
7) I lost consciousness                      YES… NO…
8) Heart beating too Fast                    YES… NO…
9) Having Heart Palpitations                 YES… NO…
10) Feeling Dizzy                            YES… NO …
11) Having Blackouts                         YES… NO…
12) This Period came too soon                YES…. NO…
13) Getting Tired easily                     YES… NO…
14) I think my HB is low                     YES… NO…
15) I Missed my Period                       YES… NO…

16) WRITE OTHER COMPLAINTS YOU MAY EXPERIENCE WHICH ARE NOT LISTED ABOVE


If you answered YES to any of the statements above, you probably lost too much blood in this cycle. It is recommended you see your doctor for check ups.

i4U

Before you go, Record the number of Pads or Tampons used in this Cycle in the Table below:

| Day of Menses | # of Standard Pads used | Or Number of Tampons used | # Improvised Pads used |
|---|---|---|---|
|  | SOAKED (x) | NOT SOAKED (y) |  |
| Day 1 |  |  |  |
| Day 2 |  |  |  |
| Day 3 |  |  |  |
| Day 4 |  |  |  |
| Day 5 |  |  |  |
| Day 6 |  |  |  |
| Day 7 |  |  |  |
|  |  |  |  |
|  | Total: | Total : |  |
|  |  |  |  |

Which of the Following Complaints did you experience 7 to 10 days before your period?

1) Breast PAIN — YES/ NO
2) Vomiting — YES/NO
3) NAUSEA — YES/NO
4) HEADACHE — YES/NO
5) DEPRESSION or Feeling Low — YES/NO
6) LOSS OF APPETITE — YES/NO
7) CONSTIPATION — YES/NO
8) BACKACHE — YES/NO
9) ANGER — YES/NO
10) IRRITABLE — YES/NO
11) AGITATION — YES/NO
12) LACK OF SELF CONTROL — YES/NO
13) DIFFICULTIES with concentration — YES/NO
14) TIREDNESS — YES/NO
15) INSOMNIA — YES/NO
16) I FEEL LUMPS IN MY BREASTS — YES/NO
17) WRITE OTHER COMPLAINTS YOU MAY EXPERIENCE WHICH ARE NOT LISTED ABOVE

If you answered YES to most of these statements, you probably experienced pre Menstrual tension or could be suffering from pre menstrual syndrome. Consult your

*i4U*

gyneacologist for advice. See a Surgeon or Nurse for advice on Lumps in Your Breast.

## *i4U - Information for you*

# Ovarian cysts before the menopause

**About this information**

This information is for you if you are premenopausal (have not gone through the menopause) and your doctor thinks you might have a cyst on one or both of your ovaries. It tells you about cysts on the ovary and the tests and treatment you may be offered.

This information aims to help you and your healthcare team make the best decisions about your care. It is not meant to replace advice from a doctor about your situation.

**What are ovaries?**

Ovaries are a woman's reproductive organs that make female hormones and release an egg from a follicle (a small fluid-filled sac) each month. The follicle is usually about 2–3 cm when measured across (diameter) but sometimes can be larger.

**What is an ovarian cyst?**

An ovarian cyst is a larger fluid-filled sac (more than 3 cm in diameter) that develops on or in an ovary. A cyst can vary in size from a few centimetres to the size of a large melon. Ovarian cysts may be thin-walled and only contain fluid (known as a simple cyst) or they may be more complex, containing thick fluid, blood or solid areas.

There are many different types of ovarian cyst that occur before the menopause, examples of which include:

- a **simple cyst**, which is usually a large follicle that has continued to grow after an egg has been released; simple cysts are the most common cysts to occur before the menopause and most disappear within a few months

- an **endometrioma** – endometriosis, where cells of the lining of the womb are found outside the womb, sometimes causes ovarian cysts and these are called endometriomas

- a **dermoid cyst**, which develops from the cells that make eggs in the ovary, often contains substances such as hair and fat.

Other types of cyst on the ovary are less common.

Almost all ovarian cysts that occur before the menopause are benign. Cancer of the ovary before the menopause is rare.

### How common are ovarian cysts?

Ovarian cysts are common. Most women will be unaware that they have a cyst as they often cause no symptoms and disappear spontaneously with time. However, up to 1 in 10 women may need surgery for an ovarian cyst at some point in their lives.

### What symptoms might I have?

Most cysts are diagnosed by chance, for example during a routine examination, or if you have an ultrasound scan for another reason. Therefore you may have no symptoms at all.

However, you may experience one or more of the following:

- lower abdominal pain or pelvic pain
- painful periods, or a change in the pattern of your periods
- pain during sex
- pain related to your bowels
- a feeling that you want to pass urine urgently and more frequently
- a change in appetite or feeling full quickly
- a distended (swollen) abdomen
- difficulty in becoming pregnant which may be linked to endometriosis.

### What happens if my doctor thinks I might have an ovarian cyst?

You will normally be asked questions about your general health, your periods, whether you have any pain in your lower abdomen, your sex life and any contraception that you may be using. You may also be asked if there is a family history of ovarian or breast cancer.

You will usually have an examination of your abdomen as well as an internal (vaginal) examination.

You should be offered an ultrasound scan to look at your ovaries. This is likely to include an abdominal scan and one through your vagina. In the majority of cases, the ultrasound scan will be normal and a cyst on the ovary will not be a cause of your symptoms.

If you do appear to have a cyst, the sonographer will check whether it is in your ovary. One in 10 suspected ovarian cysts actually involve other nearby structures, such as the fallopian tube or bowel. The scan will check the size and appearance of the cyst and look at your other ovary.

If your scan suggests that you have a complex cyst, you might be offered blood tests, which can help to determine what type of cyst it is. You do not need blood tests if a simple cyst is diagnosed.

## What happens next?

If your scan is reassuring and you have no symptoms, you may not need any treatment.

If you have symptoms or if the ultrasound has shown a large or a complex cyst, you are likely to be referred to the hospital. In the unlikely event that the tests suggest the possibility of cancer, you will be referred to a gynaecological cancer specialist for further investigation.

## What treatments might I be offered?

Treatment options include 'watching and waiting' or an operation to remove the cyst if it is getting bigger or is complex. Your choice depends on your symptoms, the appearance and the size, and the results of any blood tests. You should be given information about the choices in your individual situation, including information about the risks and benefits of each option.

## I have a simple cyst on my ovary that causes no pain – what are my options?

**A simple cyst that measures less than 5 cm in diameter** Normally, treatment is not necessary. These cysts usually disappear on their own after a few months. You are unlikely to need a follow-up appointment.

**A simple cyst that measures 5–7 cm in diameter** You should be offered follow-up, usually an ultrasound scan a year later.

**A simple cyst that measures more than 7 cm in diameter** You may be offered further tests, such as magnetic resonance imaging (MRI) and/or surgery.

## I have been advised to have surgery to remove the cyst – what type of operation will it be?

You will usually be offered laparoscopic (keyhole) surgery, which is less painful afterwards than a laparotomy (open surgery) and usually means that you can leave hospital earlier and will recover more quickly.

A laparotomy (open operation) may be recommended if the cyst is very large or, rarely, if there is a suspicion of cancer. Your gynaecologist should discuss these procedures with you, explaining the benefits and risks, and advise you which procedure is best for your situation.

**Will my ovaries be removed if I have an operation?**

Your ovaries are unlikely to be removed. The ovaries produce important hormones before the menopause and therefore in most cases only the cyst is removed.

However, there are some circumstances where the ovary may need to be removed, for example if the cyst is very large or has completely replaced the entire ovary. The ovary may also need to be removed if the cyst has twisted so much that the ovary's blood supply has been cut off, or, rarely, if there is a suspicion that the cyst may be cancerous.

Your gynaecologist should discuss the pros and cons of removing ovaries before surgery.

**What if I am pregnant and my ultrasound scan has shown that I have a cyst?**

Simple ovarian cysts are often found on the ultrasound scan during pregnancy and most will disappear as pregnancy progresses. If the cyst is large or complex, you may be offered further scans during pregnancy and a scan after your baby is born. An operation to remove the cyst during pregnancy would only be recommended if you have pain thought to be due to the cyst, or, very rarely, if cancer is suspected.

**Is there anything else I need to know?**

Taking the combined oral contraceptive pill will **not** help a simple cyst disappear although taking the pill may stop further cysts developing in the future.

Removing fluid from a simple cyst (aspiration) is of little benefit as the cyst is likely to fill up again, although it may be done to help to determine what type of cyst it is.

**Key points**

Ovarian cysts are common in women before the menopause.
Ovarian cancer is rare in women before the menopause.
An ultrasound scan should provide reassurance.
Small simple ovarian cysts usually require no treatment.

If you have surgery, this will usually be keyhole with removal of only the cyst.

**Reproduced from: Royal College of Obstetricians and Gynaecologists.** Ovarian Cysts before the menopause patient information leaflet, London, RCOG, Jun 2013, with the permission of the Royal College of Obstetricians and Gynaecologists.

i4U

## June 20......

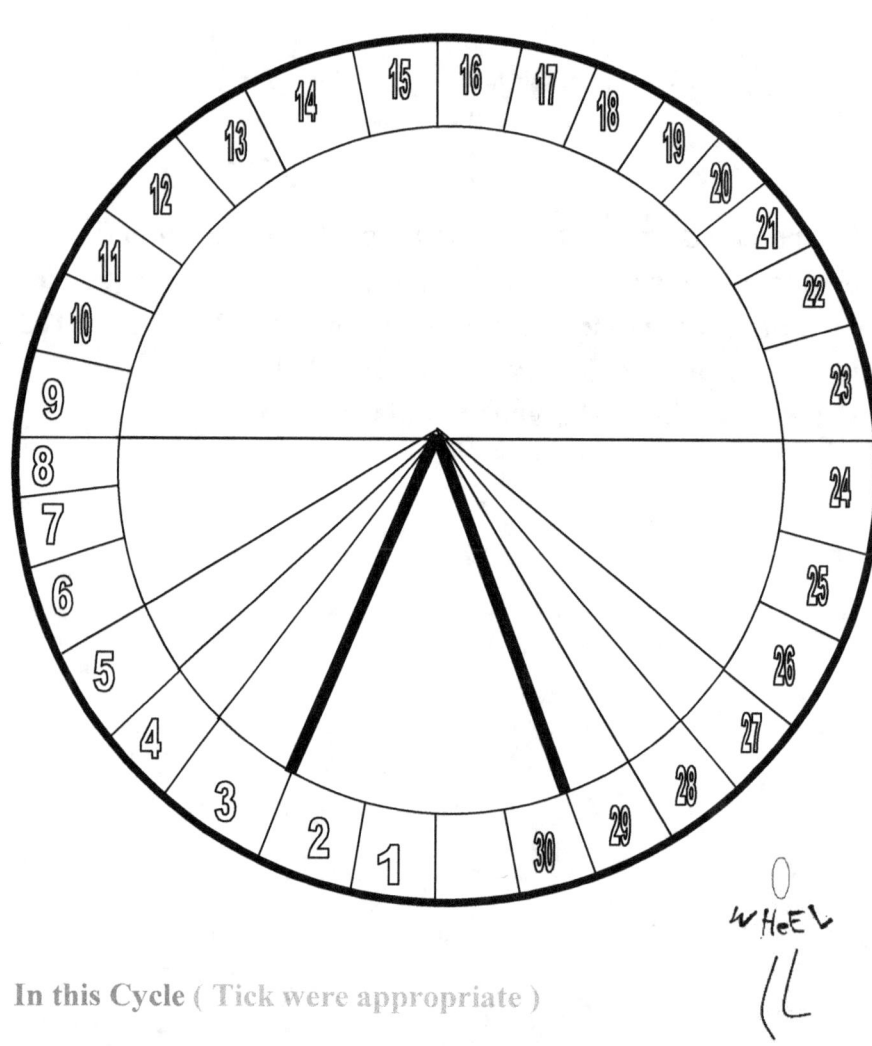

WHeEL

**In this Cycle** ( Tick were appropriate )

1) **Period lasted longer**      YES... NO...
2) **Used more pads than usual**      YES... NO...

3) Used more tampons than is usual        YES... NO...
4) I Fainted                              YES... NO...
5) More pads soaked than usual            YES... NO...
6) More tampons soaked than is usual      YES... NO...
7) Bleeding with Clots                    YES... NO...
8) Heart beating too Fast                 YES... NO...
9) Having Heart Palpitations              YES... NO...
10) My feet are getting swollen           YES... NO...
11) Having Blackouts                      YES... NO...
12) This Period came too soon             YES.... NO...
13) Getting Tired easily                  YES...NO...
14) My HB is less than 8 g/dl             YES...NO...
15) I Missed my Period                    YES...NO...
16) WRITE OTHER COMPLAINTS YOU MAY EXPERIENCE WHICH ARE NOT LISTED ABOVE

If you answered YES to any of the statements above, you probably lost too much blood in this cycle. It is recommended you see your doctor for check ups.

Before you go, Record the number of Pads or Tampons used in this Cycle in the Table below:

i4U

| Day of Menses | # of Standard Pads used | Or Number of Tampons used | # Improvised Pads used |
|---|---|---|---|
| | SOAKED (x) | NOT SOAKED (y) | |
| Day 1 | | | |
| Day 2 | | | |
| Day 3 | | | |
| Day 4 | | | |
| Day 5 | | | |
| Day 6 | | | |
| Day 7 | | | |
| | | | |
| | | | |
| | | | |

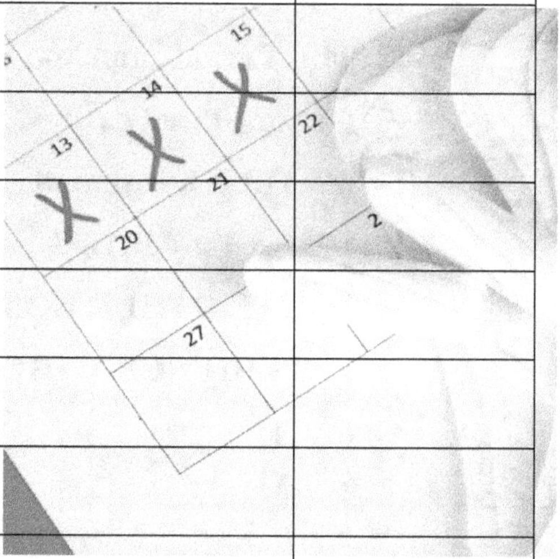

Which of the Following Complaints did you experience 7 to 10 days before your menses?

1) Breast PAIN  YES/ NO
2) Vomiting  YES/NO
3) NAUSEA  YES/NO

4) HEADACHE — YES/NO
5) DEPRESSION or Feeling Low — YES/NO
6) LOSS OF APPETITE — YES/NO
7) CONSTIPATION — YES/NO
8) BACKACHE — YES/NO
9) ANGER — YES/NO
10) IRRITABLE — YES/NO
11) AGITATION — YES/NO
12) LACK OF SELF CONTROL — YES/NO
13) DIFFICULTIES with concentration — YES/NO
14) TIREDNESS — YES/NO
15) INSOMNIA — YES/NO
16) I FEEL LUMPS IN MY BREASTS — YES/NO
17) WRITE OTHER COMPLAINTS YOU MAY EXPERIENCE WHICH ARE NOT LISTED ABOVE

If you answered YES to most of these statements, you probably experienced pre Menstrual tension or could be suffering from pre menstrual syndrome. Consult your gyneacologist for advice. See a Surgeon or Nurse for advice on Lumps in Your Breast.

SHOW THIS BOOK TO YOUR HEALTH CARE PROVIDER DURING MENSTRUAL HEALTH CONSULTATION

## i4U - Information for you

# Ovarian Cancer

**Who is this information for?**

This information is for you if you have ovarian cancer or want to know more about it. It tells you about the most common form of ovarian cancer, the stages and grades of cancer, and the treatment you may be offered. It may be helpful if you are a partner, friend or relative of someone with ovarian cancer.

Being diagnosed with ovarian cancer will be a worrying and distressing time for you and your family. The team of healthcare professionals looking after you will support you and give you information that you might find helpful. This information is to complement the support you will get.

**What is ovarian cancer and how common is it?**

Cancer is a disease of cells in the body. Normally cells grow and multiply in an orderly way, with new cells made only when they are needed. When someone has cancer, this process goes wrong and cancer cells grow and multiply too quickly. As they multiply and grow, the cancer cells damage healthy tissue.

In ovarian cancer, the cancer cells come from the ovary. This is called a primary ovarian cancer. However, in some instances these cells are thought to come from the fallopian tubes that are close to your ovaries. Sometimes the cells can spread beyond the ovary to the womb, abdomen and lungs. The cells then grow in these new sites as secondary tumours. When cancer spreads like this, it is called metastasis.

In the UK, ovarian cancer is the fifth most common cancer in women, with over 6500 women diagnosed each year. The majority of cases occur in women who have gone through the menopause and are usually aged over 50, but younger women can also be affected. The earlier the disease is found and treated, the better the survival rate.

There are several types of ovarian cancer. The most common type is epithelial ovarian cancer, which develops from the surface layer of cells in the ovary. This cancer type is rare in young women and is usually found in women who have been through the menopause.

The following information relates to epithelial ovarian cancer.

*i4U*

**What causes ovarian cancer?**

In most cases, the reason why ovarian cancer develops is unknown. However, there are factors that can affect the risk of ovarian cancer developing:

> - The risk increases with age. More than 8 out of 10 cases occur in women over the age of 50.
> - Being overweight or obese increases the risk.
> - If the number of eggs a woman releases (ovulation) during her lifetime is reduced, her risk of getting ovarian cancer is lower. Factors that reduce the number of times a woman ovulates include taking the oral contraceptive pill, being pregnant or breastfeeding. The risk increases slightly in women who have not had children and who have a late menopause.
> - A family history of ovarian or breast cancer increases the risk. This can be the result of a faulty gene. The most common faulty genes are *BRCA1* and *BRCA2*. About 1 in 10 ovarian cancers may be caused by a faulty gene. If you are concerned that you or your family may be at increased risk, talk to your specialist team or your GP who can refer you to a genetic counselling clinic for advice and testing.

**What symptoms might I have?**

Most women have very few symptoms but you may experience one or more of the following:

- lower abdominal pain or pelvic pain
- pain during sex
- pain related to your bowels
- a feeling that you want to pass urine urgently and more frequently

- a change in appetite or feeling full quickly
- a distended (swollen) abdomen.

**How is it diagnosed?**

Ovarian cancer may be suspected if an ovary appears abnormal on an ultrasound scan. Abnormal blood tests such as high levels of a protein called CA125 can make it more likely that it is malignant.

You are likely to be offered a CT scan (computed tomography scan) of your abdomen and pelvis. Sometimes you may be advised to have a biopsy (the taking of a small sample of tissue for examination). This may be done with you awake in the X-ray department or as a keyhole operation with a general anaesthetic.

If your abdomen is swollen with fluid (called ascites) you may be advised to have this drained. This is usually done under ultrasound guidance. The removed fluid may be checked for cancer cells.

If cancer is confirmed, you will be referred to a specialist gynaecology cancer centre to plan treatment.

**What are the stages and grades of the disease?**

The stage of a cancer tells you how far the cancer has spread. Doctors divide ovarian cancer into four stages. The stage can only be confirmed by having surgery.

Stage 1 – only affecting one or both of the ovaries

Stage 2 – has spread outside the ovaries but not outside the pelvis

Stage 3 – has spread outside the pelvis to the lining of the abdomen and bowel

Stage 4 – has spread to other parts of the body such as liver, spleen, lungs

Cancer cells are graded according to how they look under a microscope. The cancer can be low grade (slow-growing in appearance), moderate grade (more abnormal than low grade) or high grade (fast-growing in appearance).

The stage and grade of disease will help your specialist team decide on the best type of treatment for you.

## What are the treatment options?

Treatment options include surgery, chemotherapy and occasionally radiotherapy.

The treatment you will be offered will depend on the stage and grade of the cancer, your general health and your own wishes. You should be advised on the benefits, risks, side effects and likely success rate of treatment options. There is a good chance of successful treatment if your cancer is diagnosed at an early stage.

The team caring for you may use the word 'remission', which means there is no sign of cancer returning after treatment has ended. The more advanced the cancer is at the time of diagnosis, the less likely you will go into remission, but treatment can often shrink the cancer and relieve symptoms. New forms of treatment for ovarian cancer are being developed. Your specialist team will be able to discuss the best treatment option for your individual circumstances.

## Surgery

Most women will require surgery. The type of surgery will depend on the cancer stage and grade and on your wishes. Surgery usually involves removing both ovaries and the fallopian tubes (called a bilateral salpingo-oophorectomy), the womb and cervix (called a total hysterectomy) and the layer of fatty tissue in the abdomen known as the omentum (called an omentectomy). Biopsies and some lymph nodes may also be taken from your abdomen and pelvis. This helps to give an accurate idea of the stage the cancer has reached and to decide whether you need further treatment.

If the cancer has spread to other areas of your pelvis or abdomen, your surgeon will remove as much of the cancer as safely possible.

The less cancer left in your body after surgery, the more likely chemotherapy is to work.

If the cancer is at an early stage and you wish to become pregnant, you may only need to have the affected ovary and tube removed. Your specialist team will discuss with you the benefits and risks of this form of surgery and they will also discuss the possibility of egg or embryo freezing before treatment.

Surgery may not always be possible because of where the cancer is or if you are not well enough for an operation. If this is the case, your specialist team may recommend chemotherapy to shrink the tumour and relieve symptoms.

**Chemotherapy**

Chemotherapy treats cancer by using anti-cancer (cytotoxic) drugs to kill cancer cells. Ovarian cancer is usually very sensitive to chemotherapy. It is usually given after surgery. Sometimes it may be given before surgery, usually to help shrink the tumour and to make it easier to remove. This is called neoadjuvant chemotherapy.

There are a number of different anti-cancer drugs and different treatment plans. You may have a single drug or a combination of drugs. The choice of drug and how and when it is given depends on the stage and grade of your cancer and your general health. You are most likely to have either a platinum-containing drug (carboplatin) on its own or in combination with another anti-cancer drug called paclitaxel.

You will usually be given the chemotherapy through a drip in your arm over several hours in hospital. Most women have the treatment as an outpatient. A session of chemotherapy is followed by a period of rest to allow your body to recover. This is known as a cycle and often takes 3 weeks. Most women have six cycles of chemotherapy.

There are some side effects of chemotherapy. These will depend on the drugs you have, the dose and your individual reaction to the drug.

The main side effects of chemotherapy are caused by its effect on the healthy cells in your body. Side effects may include nausea and vomiting, loss of appetite, tiredness, a sore mouth, hair loss, numbness or tingling in the hands and feet, and an increased risk of getting infections. Often these side effects can be well controlled with medication.

**Radiotherapy**

Radiotherapy is a treatment that uses high-energy radiation beams to target rapidly growing cancer cells. Radiotherapy is not often used in the treatment of ovarian cancer but your specialist team may recommend it in some circumstances such as for shrinking a secondary tumour and/or for treatment of pain.

**Supportive care**

You may not be well enough to have the treatment/s described above or you may decide against anti-cancer treatment. If so, you should discuss your wishes with your healthcare professionals. You will be offered treatment to relieve symptoms. This is known as supportive or palliative care.

**How will I know whether the treatment is working?**

As well as clinical follow-up by your doctor, the following may be helpful to monitor your response to treatment:

- CA125 blood test – in response to treatment, the level of CA125 will gradually fall and return to a normal value
- imaging scans such as chest X-rays or CT or MRI (magnetic resonance imaging) scans – these techniques will look for signs of cancer in your pelvis, abdomen and chest.

**What are the treatment options if the cancer returns?**

Cancer can return after treatment. If this happens, you are likely to be offered another course of chemotherapy. There are a number of anti-cancer drugs that can be used. Your specialist will recommend the drug or drug combination that is best for you. This will depend on the type of ovarian cancer, the drugs you had before and how well they worked, how long you were in remission and what side effects you had. You may be advised to have carboplatin again, usually in combination with another drug such as gemcitabine.

**Targeted therapies**

These are new types of cancer treatment. By targeting a particular part of the tumour cell, these drugs may cause less damage to healthy cells than more traditional chemotherapy. The benefits of drugs that stop the formation of new blood vessels, such as bevacizumab, used in combination with other chemotherapy drugs are still being tested. If your specialist recommends bevacizumab, he or she will explain why as well as discuss the possible side effects.

If you have developed ovarian cancer due to a faulty *BRCA1* or *BRCA2* gene, you may be treated with drugs called PARP inhibitors. These drugs target tumour cells while sparing normal cells. The benefits of these drugs are still being assessed and tested.

If you are asked to take part in a clinical trial on the treatment of ovarian cancer, you will be given written and verbal information so you can make an informed decision on whether or not to take part. If you do not wish to take part or if you withdraw from the trial at any stage, this will not affect the quality of the care you will receive.5

*i4U*

**Follow-up after treatment**

Your specialist team will advise you to have regular hospital follow-ups after treatment. For the first couple of years you will have follow-up appointments every 2–3 months. If all remains well, the visits will then become less frequent and you may only be seen once or twice a year for up to 5 years.

It is important to attend these follow-up visits even if you are feeling well, as cancer can return even when you have no symptoms. Should you get symptoms or be worried about anything, contact your GP or your specialist team as soon as possible. Do not wait until your next appointment.

At your follow-up visit, the doctor will ask you how you are feeling and whether you have any symptoms or are suffering from side effects of treatment. He or she will usually examine you. You may also have blood tests, scans or X-rays to see how your cancer has responded to treatment.

**Support during and after treatment**

Coping with cancer can be emotionally challenging. Your specialist team and your GP will help and support both you and your family. You should be offered contact details for a key worker who is often a clinical nurse specialist. Don't be afraid to ask questions, to talk about your feelings and to ask for help. You may find it beneficial to see a trained counsellor. You may also find it helpful to talk to someone else who has also had ovarian cancer and treatment.

If your ovaries have been removed before your menopause, you may want to consider hormone replacement therapy (HRT). You should talk to your specialist team about this.

**Reproduced from: Royal College of Obstetricians and Gynaecologists. Ovarian Cancer patient information leaflet, London, RCOG, Jan 2016, with the permission**

of the Royal College of Obstetricians and Gynaecologists

i4U

July                                  20......

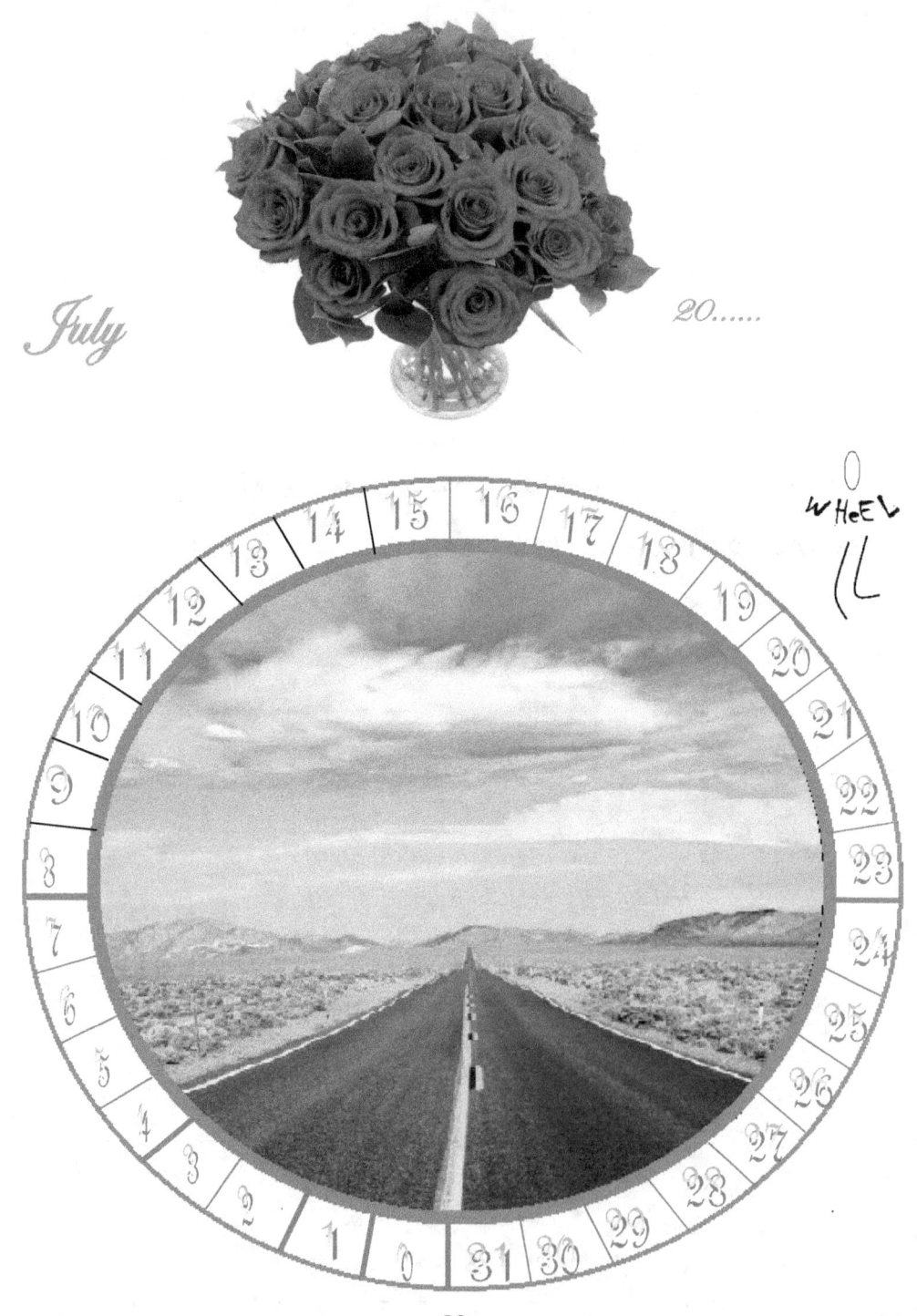

WHeEL

In the July Menstrual Cycle ( Tick were appropriate )

1) Period lasted longer                           YES… NO…
2) Used more pads than is usual for me            YES… NO…
3) Used more tampons than is usual               YES… NO…
4) **I COULDN'T WORK**                            YES… NO…
5) More pads soaked than is usual                 YES… NO…
6) More tampons soaked than is usual              YES… NO…
7) Bleeding with Clots                            YES… NO…
8) Heart beating too Fast                         YES… NO…
9) Having Heart Palpitations                      YES… NO…
10) Feeling Dizzy                                 YES… NO …
11) Having Blackouts                              YES… NO…
12) This Period came too soon                     YES…. NO…
13) Getting Tired easily                          YES…NO…
14) My HB is less than 8 g/dl                     YES…NO…
15) I Missed my Period                            YES…NO…
16) **WRITE OTHER COMPLAINTS YOU MAY EXPERIENCE WHICH ARE NOT LISTED ABOVE**

If you answered YES to any of the statements above, you probably lost too much blood in this cycle. It is recommended you see your doctor for check ups.

Before you go, Record the number of Pads or Tampons used in this Cycle in the Table below:

| Day of Menses | # of Standard Pads used | Or Number of Tampons used | # Improvised Pads used |
|---|---|---|---|
| | SOAKED (x) | NOT SOAKED (y) | |
| Day 1 | | | |
| Day 2 | | | |
| Day 3 | | | |
| Day 4 | | | |
| Day 5 | | | |
| Day 6 | | | |
| Day 7 | | | |
| | | | |
| | Total: | Total : | |
| | | | |

Which of the Following Complaints did you experience 7 to 10 days before your menses?

| | |
|---|---|
| 1) Breast PAIN | YES/NO |
| 2) Vomiting | YES/NO |
| 3) NAUSEA | YES/NO |
| 4) HEADACHE | YES/NO |
| 5) DEPRESSION or Feeling Low | YES/NO |
| 6) LOSS OF APPETITE | YES/NO |
| 7) CONSTIPATION | YES/NO |
| 8) BACKACHE | YES/NO |
| 9) ANGER | YES/NO |
| 10) IRRITABLE | YES/NO |
| 11) AGITATION | YES/NO |
| 12) LACK OF SELF CONTROL | YES/NO |
| 13) DIFFICULTIES with concentration | YES/NO |
| 14) TIREDNESS | YES/NO |
| 15) INSOMNIA | YES/NO |
| 16) I FEEL LUMPS IN MY BREASTS | YES/NO |

17) WRITE OTHER COMPLAINTS YOU MAY EXPERIENCE WHICH ARE NOT LISTED ABOVE

If you answered YES to most of these statements, you probably experienced pre Menstrual tension or could be suffering from Pre Menstrual Syndrome (PMS). Consult your gyneacologist for advice. See a Surgeon or Nurse for advice on Lumps in Your Breast.

*i4U*

# *i4U – Information for you*

## Acute pelvic inflammatory disease

This information is for you if you want to know more about acute pelvic inflammatory disease (PID), how it is diagnosed and how it is treated. It may also be helpful if you are a relative or friend of someone who has this condition.

**What is pelvic inflammatory disease?**

PID is an inflammation of the pelvic organs. It is usually caused by an infection spreading from the vagina and cervix to the uterus (womb), fallopian tubes, ovaries and pelvic area. If severe, it can cause an abscess (collection of pus) inside the pelvis.

PID is common and accounts for one in 60 GP visits by women under the age of 45 years. **What is 'acute' pelvic inflammatory disease?** Acute PID is when there is sudden or severe inflammation of the uterus, fallopian tubes, ovaries and pelvic area due to infection. The inflammation can persist for a long time; this is known as chronic pelvic inflammatory disease (see **Are there any long-term effects?**). 45years.**What is 'acute' pelvic inflammatory disease?** Acute PID is when there is sudden or severe inflammation of the uterus, fallopian tubes, ovaries and pelvic area due to infection. Sometimes the inflammation can persist for a long time; this is known as chronic pelvic inflammatory disease.

**What is 'acute' pelvic inflammatory disease?**

Acute PID is inflammation of the uterus, fallopian tubes, ovaries and pelvic area caused by an infection. If left untreated, it can cause abdominal pain and fertility problems in the future.

Sometimes the inflammation can persist for a long time and this is known as chronic PID (see the section 'Are there any long-term effects?').

**What causes it?**

Untreated sexually transmitted infections (STIs) such as chlamydia or gonorrhoea are the most likely causes of PID and account for one-quarter of the cases in the UK.

PID may also be caused by a number of less common infections that may, or may not, be sexually transmitted. Acute PID is more common in young, sexually active women.

Occasionally, PID can develop after a miscarriage or termination of pregnancy, after having a baby or after a procedure such as insertion of an intrauterine device (IUD) or coil.

## What are the symptoms?

Sometimes you may not have any obvious symptoms. You may have one or more of the following, which can vary from mild to severe:

- smelly or unusual vaginal discharge
- pain in the lower abdomen that is usually on both sides and can feel like period pains
- pain deep inside during or after sex
- vaginal bleeding in between periods, bleeding after sex, or heavy periods
- nausea and vomiting
- fever
- low backache.

Many of these symptoms are common and can be caused by other conditions.

This means that PID can be difficult to diagnose so, if you have any of these symptoms, it is important to seek medical advice as soon as possible.

## How is it diagnosed?

Your doctor will ask you about your symptoms and your medical and sexual history. With your consent, your doctor may also do a vaginal (internal) examination. You should be offered a female chaperone for this. The examination may cause some discomfort, especially if you do have PID.

Swabs may be taken from your vagina and your cervix to test for infection. It usually takes a few days for the results to come back.

a **positive** swab result confirms that you do have an infection a **negative** swab result, however, does not mean you are definitely clear of infection.

Sometimes an additional swab may be taken from the urethra (the tube through which urine empties out of your bladder). This can make it easier to detect chlamydia and gonorrhoea or other infections.

**Further tests**

You may be offered blood tests to check for infection. You may be asked for a urine sample. A test for HIV may also be advised.

If there is a chance that you could be pregnant, you will be offered a pregnancy test. This is because other conditions such as ectopic pregnancy (when a pregnancy develops outside the womb) can cause similar symptoms to PID.

If your doctor suspects you have a severe infection, you will be referred to your local hospital for further tests and treatment. You may be offered:

- an ultrasound scan. This is usually a transvaginal scan (where a probe is gently inserted into your vagina) to look more closely at the uterus (womb), fallopian tubes and ovaries. This may help to detect inflamed fallopian tubes or an abscess.
- an operation under a general anaesthetic called a laparoscopy, which is sometimes called keyhole surgery. The doctor uses a small telescope called a laparoscope to look at your pelvis by making tiny cuts, usually into your umbilicus (tummy button) and just above the bikini line. Laparoscopy can help diagnose PID and can be used to drain a pelvic abscess.

**What is the treatment?**

Your doctor or nurse can give you information about the specific treatment you are offered; this should include information about possible side effects.

*i4U*

You will usually be given an injection of an antibiotic followed by a 2 week course of antibiotic tablets. Treatment usually does not interfere with contraception or pregnancy. It is very important to complete your course of antibiotics even if you are feeling better. Most women who complete the course have no long-term health or fertility problems.

You may also be offered medication for pain relief. You should rest until your symptoms improve. If they get worse, or do not get better within 48 to 72 hours of treatment, you should see your doctor again.

**When does treatment start?**

You should start taking antibiotics as soon as they are prescribed, even if you have not had your test results back. This is because any delay could increase the risk of long-term health problems (see the section 'Are there any long-term effects?').

**Why might I need hospital treatment?**

Your doctor may recommend treatment in hospital if:

- your diagnosis is unclear
- you are very unwell
- they suspect an abscess in your fallopian tube and/or ovary
- you are pregnant
- you are not getting better within a few days of starting oral antibiotics
- you are unable to take antibiotic tablets.

When you are in hospital, antibiotics may be given intravenously (directly into the blood stream through a drip). This treatment is usually continued until 24 hours after your symptoms have improved. After that, you will also be given a course of antibiotic tablets.

**Will I need an operation?**

You will usually only need an operation if you have a severe infection or an abscess in the fallopian tube and/or ovary. An abscess may be drained during a laparoscopy or during an ultrasound procedure. The doctor will discuss these treatments with you in greater detail.

**What if I'm pregnant?**

It is rare to develop PID when you are pregnant.

If there is any chance you could be pregnant, you should tell your doctor or nurse as certain antibiotics should be avoided in pregnancy. The risks that are associated with the type of antibiotics prescribed for PID are low for both mother and baby.

**What if I have an intrauterine contraceptive device (IUD/coil)?**

If your symptoms of PID are not improving within a few days of starting treatment and you have an IUD, your doctor may recommend that you have it removed. If you have had sex in the 7 days before it is removed, you will be at risk of pregnancy, and emergency hormonal contraception (the morning-after pill) may be offered.

**Should my partner be treated?**

If you have developed PID as a result of an STI, anyone you have had sex with in the last 6 months should be tested for infection, even if they are well. You can contact them yourself or, your doctor, local genitourinary medicine (GUM) clinic or sexual health clinic may help you with this.

## When can I have sex again?

You should avoid having any sexual contact for 1 week after both you and your partner have completed the course of treatment, to avoid re-infection.

## What about follow-up?

If you have a moderate to severe infection, you will usually be given an appointment to return to the clinic after 3 days. It is important to attend this appointment so that your doctor can see that your symptoms are responding to the antibiotics.

If your symptoms are not improving, you may be advised to attend hospital for further investigations and treatment.

If your symptoms are improving, you will usually be given a further follow-up appointment 4 to 6 weeks later to check:

- that your treatment has been effective
- whether a repeat swab test is needed to confirm that the infection has been successfully treated; this is particularly important if you have ongoing symptoms
- that you have all the information you need about the long-term effects of PID
- whether another pregnancy test is needed
- that you have all the information you need about future contraceptive choices
- that your sexual partner(s) have been treated.

## Are there any long-term effects?

Treatment with antibiotics is usually successful for acute PID. Long-term problems can arise if it is untreated, if treatment is delayed, or if there is a severe infection.

The long-term effects can be:

> ➢ scarring of the fallopian tube, which can cause: an increased risk of ectopic pregnancy difficulties in becoming pregnant

> ➢ an abscess in a fallopian tube and/or ovary

> ➢ persistent pain in your lower abdomen;

See the RCOG patient information *Chronic (long-term) pelvic pain.* Repeated episodes of PID increase the risk of future fertility problems. Risks of further infection can be reduced by using condoms and by making sure that you and your sexual partner(s) have been treated.

**Key points**

- Pelvic inflammatory disease (PID) is an inflammation of the pelvic organs.

- Diagnosis is usually based on symptoms, examination and test results.

- Acute PID is usually treated successfully with antibiotics. Rarely, surgical treatment may be required.

- It is advisable to avoid having any sexual contact until you and your partner have completed the course of treatment and follow-up.

**Reproduced from: Royal College of Obstetricians and Gynaecologists. Acute Pelvic Inflammatory disease**

*i4U*

patient information leaflet, London, RCOG, Nov 2016, with the permission of the Royal College of Obstetricians and Gynaecologists

# August 20......

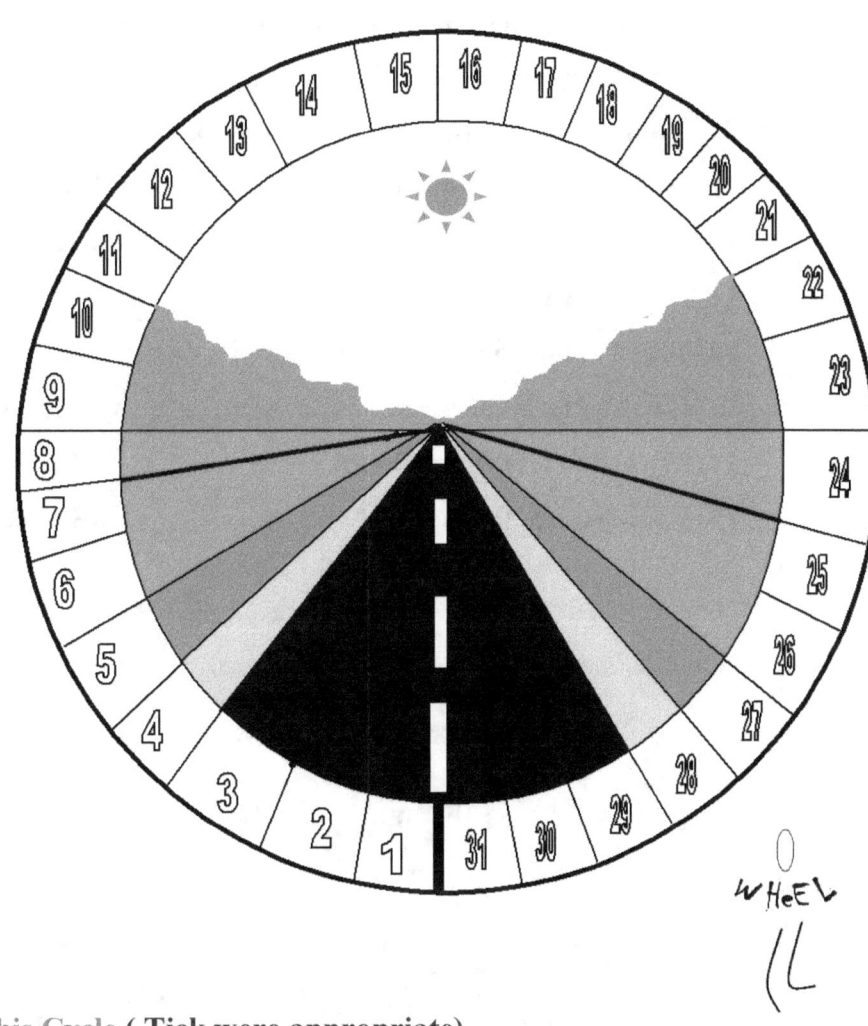

In this Cycle ( Tick were appropriate)

1) Period lasted longer than seven days    YES... NO...
2) Used more pads than is usual for me    YES... NO...

*i4U*

3) Used more tampons than is usual    YES... NO...
4) I was admitted to hospital    YES... NO...
5) More pads soaked than is usual    YES... NO...
6) More tampons soaked than is usual    YES... NO...
7) Bleeding with Clots    YES... NO...
8) Having severe abdominal & back pain    YES... NO...
9) Having Heart Palpitations    YES... NO...
10) Having nose bleeds    YES... NO ...
11) Having Blackouts    YES... NO...
12) This Period came too soon    YES.... NO...
13) Getting Tired easily    YES...NO...
14) My HB is less than 10 g/dl    YES...NO...
15) I Missed my Period    YES...NO...

If you answered YES to any of the statements above, you probably lost too much blood in this cycle. It is recommended you see your doctor for check ups.

Before you go, Record the number of Pads or Tampons used in this Cycle in the Table below:

| Day of Menses | # of Standard Pads used | Or Number of Tampons used | # Improvised Pads used |
|---|---|---|---|
| | SOAKED (x) | NOT SOAKED (y) | |

|  |  |  |  |
|---|---|---|---|
| Day 1 |  |  |  |
| Day 2 |  |  |  |
| Day 3 |  |  |  |
| Day 4 |  |  |  |
| Day 5 |  |  |  |
| Day 6 |  |  |  |
| Day 7 |  |  |  |
|  |  |  |  |
|  | Total: | Total : |  |
|  |  |  |  |

Which of the Following Complaints did you experience 7 to 10 days before your menses?

1) **Breast PAIN** — YES/ NO
2) **Vomiting** — YES/NO
3) **NAUSEA** — YES/NO
4) **HEADACHE** — YES/NO
5) **DEPRESSION or Feeling Low** — YES/NO
6) **LOSS OF APPETITE** — YES/NO
7) **CONSTIPATION** — YES/NO
8) **BACKACHE** — YES/NO

i4U

| | |
|---|---|
| 9) ANGER | YES/NO |
| 10) IRRITABLE | YES/NO |
| 11) AGITATION | YES/NO |
| 12) LACK OF SELF CONTROL | YES/NO |
| 13) DIFFICULTIES with concentration | YES/NO |
| 14) TIREDNESS | YES/NO |
| 15) INSOMNIA | YES/NO |
| 16) LUMPS IN MY BREASTS | YES/NO |

17) WRITE OTHER COMPLAINTS YOU MAY EXPERIENCE WHICH ARE NOT LISTED ABOVE

If you answered YES to most of these statements, you probably experienced pre Menstrual tension or could be suffering from pre menstrual syndrome. Consult your gyneacologist for advice. See a SURGEON or Nurse for advice on Lumps in Your Breast.

*i4U – Information for you*

## 3rd or 4th Degree tear during child birth

### About this information

This information is for you if you want to know more about third- or fourth-degree perineal tears (also known as obstetric anal sphincter injury – OASI). It may be helpful if you are a relative or friend of someone who is in this situation.

### What is a perineal tear?

Many women experience tears to some extent during childbirth as the baby stretches the vagina. Most tears occur in the perineum, the area between the vaginal opening and the anus (back passage).

Small, skin-deep tears are known as first-degree tears and usually heal naturally. Tears that are deeper and affect the muscle of the perineum are known as second-degree tears. These usually require stitches.

An episiotomy is a cut made by a doctor or midwife through the vaginal wall and perineum to make more space to deliver the baby.

### What is a third- or fourth-degree tear?

For some women the tear may be deeper. A tear that also involves the muscle that controls the anus (the anal sphincter) is known as a third-degree tear. If the tear extends further into the lining of the anus or rectum it is known as a fourth-degree tear.

## How common are third- or fourth-degree tears?

Overall, a third- or fourth-degree tear occurs in about 3 in 100 women having a vaginal birth. It is slightly more common with a first vaginal birth, occurring in 6 in 100 women, compared with 2 in 100 women who have had a vaginal birth previously.

## What increases my risk of a third- or fourth-degree tear?

These types of tears usually occur unexpectedly during birth and most of the time it is not possible to predict when it will happen. However, it is more likely if:

- this is your first vaginal birth
- you are of South Asian origin
- your second stage of labour (the time from when the cervix is fully dilated to birth) is longer than expected.
- you require forceps or a ventouse to help the delivery of your baby one of the baby's shoulders becomes stuck behind your pubic bone, delaying the birth of the baby's body, which is known as shoulder dystocia
- you have a large baby (over 4 kg or 8 pounds and 13 ounces)
- you have had a third- or fourth-degree tear before.

## Could anything have been done to prevent this type of tear?

In most instances, a third- or fourth-degree tear cannot be prevented because it cannot be predicted. However, applying a warm compress to the perineum while you are pushing does appear to reduce the chance of a third- or fourth-degree tear. Your midwife or obstetrician may protect the perineum as your baby's head is delivering and this may also help prevent a tear.

It is unclear whether an episiotomy will prevent a third- or fourth-degree tear from occurring during a normal vaginal birth. An episiotomy will only be performed if necessary, and with your consent.

If you have an assisted birth (ventouse or forceps), you are more likely to have an episiotomy as it may reduce the chance of a third- or fourth-degree tear occurring.

**What will happen if I have a third- or fourth-degree tear?**

If a third- or fourth-degree tear is suspected or confirmed, this will usually be repaired in the operating theatre. Your doctor will talk to you about this and you will be asked to sign a consent form. You will need an epidural or a spinal anaesthetic, although occasionally a general anaesthetic may be necessary.

You may need a drip in your arm to give you fluids until you feel able to eat and drink. You are likely to need a catheter (tube) in your bladder to drain your urine. This is usually kept in until you are able to walk to the toilet.

After the operation you will be:

- Offered pain-relieving drugs such as paracetamol, ibuprofen or diclofenac to relieve any pain.
- advised to take a course of antibiotics to reduce the risk of infection because the stitches are very close to the anus
- advised to take laxatives to make it easier and more comfortable to open your bowels.

Once you have opened your bowels and your stitches have been checked to see that they are healing properly, you should be able to go home.

### Will I be able to breastfeed?

Yes. None of the treatments offered will prevent you from breastfeeding.

### What can I expect afterwards?

After having any tear or an episiotomy, it is normal to feel pain or soreness around the tear or cut for two to three weeks after giving birth, particularly when walking or sitting. Passing urine can also cause stinging. Continue to take your painkillers when you go home.

Most of the stitches are dissolvable and the tear or cut should heal within a few weeks, although this can take longer. The stitches can irritate as healing takes place but this is normal. You may notice some stitch material fall out, which is also normal.

To start with, some women feel that they pass wind more easily or need to rush to the toilet to open their bowels. Most women make a good recovery, particularly if the tear is recognised and repaired at the time: 6–8 in 10 women will have no symptoms a year after birth.

### What can help me recover?

Keep the area clean. Have a bath or a shower at least once a day and change your sanitary pads regularly (wash your hands both before and after you do so). This will reduce the risk of infection.

You should drink at least 2–3 litres of water every day and eat a healthy balanced diet (fruit, vegetables, cereals, wholemeal bread and pasta). This will ensure that your bowels open regularly and will prevent you from becoming constipated.

Strengthening the muscles around the vagina and anus by doing pelvic floor exercises can help healing. It is important to do pelvic floor exercises as soon as you can after birth. You should be offered physiotherapy advice about pelvic floor exercises to do after surgery.

Looking after a newborn baby and recovering from an operation for a perineal tear can be hard. Support from family and friends can help.

**When should I seek medical advice after I go home?**

You should contact your midwife or general practitioner if:

- Your stitches become more painful or smelly – this may be a sign of an infection
- You cannot control your bowels or flatus (passing wind).

Talk to your GP if you have any other worries or concerns. You can be referred back to the hospital before your follow-up appointment if you wish.

**When can I have sex?**

In the weeks after having a vaginal birth, many women feel sore, whether they've had a tear or not. If you have had a tear, sex can be uncomfortable for longer. You should wait to have sex until the bleeding has stopped and the tear has healed. This may take several weeks. After that you can have sex when you feel ready to do so.

A small number of women have difficulty having sex and continue to find it painful. Talk to your doctor if this is the case so that you can get the help and support you need.4

It is possible to conceive a few weeks after your baby is born, even before you have a period. You may wish to talk with your GP or midwife about contraception or visit your local family planning clinic to discuss this.

### Your follow-up appointment

You may be offered a follow-up appointment at the hospital 6–12 weeks after you have had your baby to check that your stitches have healed properly. You will be asked questions about whether you have any problems controlling your bowels. You may be referred to a specialist if you do.

You will also have the opportunity to discuss the birth and any concerns that you may have.

### Can I have a vaginal birth in the future?

Most women go on to have a straightforward birth after a third- or fourth-degree tear.

However, there is an increased risk of this happening again in a future pregnancy. Between 5 and 7 in 100 women who have had a third- or fourth-degree tear will have a similar tear in a future pregnancy.

You may wish to consider a vaginal delivery if you have recovered well and do not have any symptoms. If you continue to experience symptoms from the third- or fourth-degree tear, you may wish to consider a planned caesarean section.

You will be able to discuss your options for future births at your follow-up appointment or early in your next pregnancy. Your individual circumstances and preferences will be taken into account.

**Reproduced from: Royal College of Obstetricians and Gynaecologists. A third or fourth degree tear during birth patient information leaflet, London, RCOG, Jun 2015, with the permission of the Royal College of Obstetricians and Gynaecologist**

*September 20......*

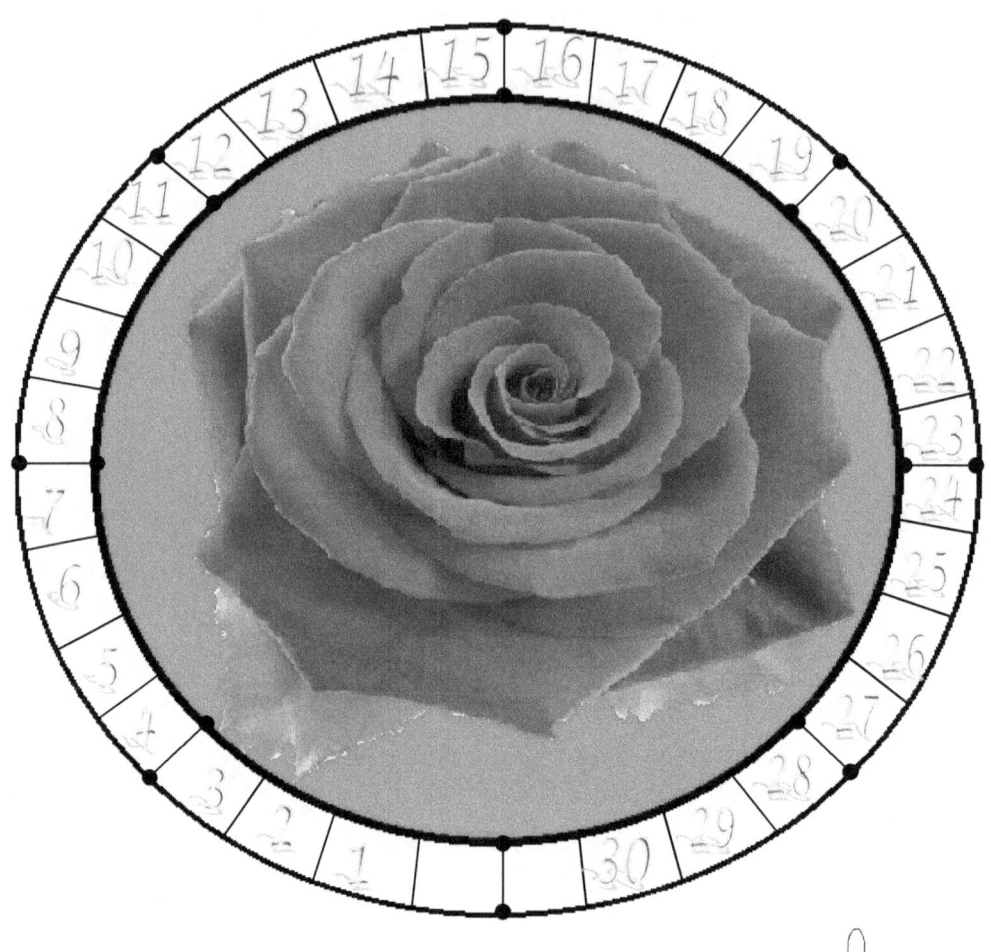

WHeEL

**In this Cycle ( Tick were appropriate )**

1) Period lasted longer than seven days     YES... NO...
2) Used more pads than is usual for me     YES... NO...
3) Used more tampons than is usual     YES... NO...

4) I Nearly Died                                    YES... NO...
5) More pads soaked than is usual                   YES... NO...
6) More tampons soaked than is usual                YES... NO...
7) Bleeding with Clots                              YES... NO...
8) Bleeding at the Umbilicus                        YES... NO...
9) Having Heart Palpitations                        YES... NO...
10) My Palms & Gums Look pale                       YES... NO ...
11) My Friends are saying I am Aneamic              YES... NO...
12) This Period came too soon                       YES.... NO...
13) Getting Tired easily                            YES...NO...
14) My HB is less than 6 g/dl                       YES...NO...
15) I Missed my Period                              YES...NO...
16) WRITE OTHER COMPLAINTS YOU MAY EXPERIENCE WHICH ARE NOT LISTED ABOVE

If you answered YES to any of the statements above, you probably lost too much blood in this cycle. It is recommended you see your doctor for check ups.

Before you go, Record the number of Pads or Tampons used in this Cycle in the table below:

| Day of | # of Standard | Or Number of Tampons used | # Improvised Pads used |
|---|---|---|---|

i4U

| Menses | Pads used | | |
|---|---|---|---|
| | SOAKED (x) | NOT SOAKED (y) | |
| Day 1 | | | |
| Day 2 | | | |
| Day 3 | | | |
| Day 4 | | | |
| Day 5 | | | |
| Day 6 | | | |
| Day 7 | | | |
| | | | |
| | Total: | Total : | |
| | | | |

Which of the Following Complaints did you experience 7 to 10 days before your menses?

1) Breast PAIN        YES/ NO
2) Vomiting           YES/NO
3) NAUSEA             YES/NO

| | |
|---|---|
| 4) HEADACHE | YES/NO |
| 5) DEPRESSION or Feeling Low | YES/NO |
| 6) LOSS OF APPETITE | YES/NO |
| 7) CONSTIPATION | YES/NO |
| 8) BACKACHE | YES/NO |
| 9) ANGER | YES/NO |
| 10) IRRITABLE | YES/NO |
| 11) AGITATION | YES/NO |
| 12) LACK OF SELF CONTROL | YES/NO |
| 13) DIFFICULTIES with concentration | YES/NO |
| 14) TIREDNESS | YES/NO |
| 15) INSOMNIA | YES/NO |
| 16) I FEEL LUMPS IN MY BREASTS | YES/NO |

17) WRITE OTHER COMPLAINTS YOU MAY EXPERIENCE WHICH ARE NOT LISTED ABOVE

If you answered YES to most of these statements, you probably experienced pre Menstrual tension or could be suffering from pre menstrual syndrome. Consult your gyneacologist for advice. See a Surgeon or Nurse for advice on Lumps in Your Breast.

*i4U – Information for you*

# Pre-eclampsia

**What is pre-eclampsia?**

Pre-eclampsia is a condition that typically occurs after 20 weeks of pregnancy. It is a combination of:

> - raised blood pressure (hypertension)
> - protein in your urine (proteinuria).

The exact cause of pre-eclampsia is not understood.

Often there are no symptoms and it may be picked up at your routine antenatal appointments when you have your blood pressure checked and urine tested. This is why you are asked to bring a urine sample to your appointments.

**Why do I need to know if I have pre-eclampsia?**

Pre-eclampsia is common, affecting between two and eight in 100 women during pregnancy. It is usually mild and normally has very little effect on pregnancy. However, it is important to know if you have the condition because, in a small number of cases, it can develop into a more serious illness. Severe pre-eclampsia can be life-threatening for both mother and baby.

Around one in 200 women (0.5%) develop severe pre-eclampsia during pregnancy. The symptoms tend to occur later on in pregnancy but can also occur for the first time only after birth.

The symptoms of severe pre-eclampsia include:

- severe headache that doesn't go away with simple painkillers

- problems with vision, such as blurring or flashing before the eyes

➢ severe pain just below the ribs

➢ heartburn that doesn't go away with antacids

➢ rapidly increasing swelling of the face, hands or feet

➢ feeling very unwell.

These symptoms are serious and you should seek medical help immediately. If in doubt, contact the maternity unit at your local hospital.

In severe pre-eclampsia, other organs, such as the liver or kidneys, can sometimes become affected and there can be problems with blood clotting.

Severe pre-eclampsia may progress to convulsions or seizures before or just after the baby's birth. These seizures are called eclamptic fits and are rare, occurring in only one in 4000 pregnancies.

**How may pre-eclampsia affect my baby?**

Pre-eclampsia affects the development of the placenta (afterbirth), which may prevent your baby growing as it should. There may also be less fluid around your baby in the womb.

If the placenta is severely affected, your baby may become very unwell. In some cases, the baby may even die in the womb. Monitoring aims to pick up those babies who are most at risk.

**Who is at risk of pre-eclampsia and can it be prevented?**

Pre-eclampsia can occur in any pregnancy but you are at higher risk if:

- your blood pressure was high before you became pregnant
- your blood pressure was high in a previous pregnancy
- you have a medical problem such as kidney problems or diabetes or a condition that affects the immune system, such as lupus.

If any of these apply to you, you should be advised to take low-dose aspirin (75 mg) once a day from 12 weeks of pregnancy, to reduce your risk.

The importance of other factors is less clear-cut, but you are more likely to develop pre-eclampsia if more than one of the following applies:

- this is your first pregnancy
- you are aged 40 or over
- your last pregnancy was more than 10 years ago
- you are very overweight – a BMI (body mass index) of 35 or more
- your mother or sister had pre-eclampsia during pregnancy
- you are carrying more than one baby.

If you have more than one of these risk factors, you may also be advised to take low-dose aspirin once a day from 12 weeks of pregnancy.

**How is pre-eclampsia monitored?**

If you are diagnosed with pre-eclampsia, you should attend hospital for assessment.

While you are at the hospital, your blood pressure will be measured regularly and you may be offered medication to help lower it. Your urine will be tested to measure the amount of protein it contains and you will also have blood tests done. Your baby's heart rate will be monitored and you may have ultrasound scans to measure your baby's growth and wellbeing.

**What happens next?**

You will continue to be monitored closely to check that you can safely carry on with your pregnancy. This may be done on an outpatient basis if you have mild pre-eclampsia. You are likely to be advised to have your baby at about 37 weeks of pregnancy, or earlier if there are concerns about you or your baby. This may mean you will need to have labour induced or, if you are having a caesarean section, to have it earlier than planned.

**What happens if I develop severe pre-eclampsia?**

If you develop severe pre-eclampsia, you will be cared for by a specialist team. The only way to prevent serious complications is for your baby to be born. Each pregnancy is unique and the exact timing will depend on your own particular situation. This should be discussed with you. There may be enough time to induce your labour. In some cases, the birth will need to be by caesarean section.

Treatment includes medication (either tablets or via a drip) to lower and control your blood pressure. You will also be given medication to prevent eclamptic fits if your baby is expected to be born within the next 24 hours or if you have experienced an eclamptic fit.

You will be closely monitored on the labour ward. In more serious cases, you may need to be admitted to an intensive care or high dependency unit.

## What happens after the birth?

Pre-eclampsia usually goes away after birth. However, if you have severe pre-eclampsia, complications may still occur within the first few days and so you will continue to be monitored closely. You may need to continue taking medication to lower your blood pressure.

If your baby has been born early or is smaller than expected, he or she may need to be monitored. There is no reason why you should not breastfeed should you wish to do so.

You may need to stay in hospital for several days. When you go home, you will be advised on how often to get your blood pressure checked and for how long to take your medication.

You should have a follow-up with your GP 6–8 weeks after birth for a final blood pressure and urine check.

If you had severe pre-eclampsia or eclampsia, you should have a postnatal appointment with your obstetrician to discuss the condition and what happened. If you are still on medication to treat your blood pressure 6 weeks after the birth, or there is still protein in your urine on testing, you may be referred to a specialist.

## Will I get pre-eclampsia in a future pregnancy?

Overall, one in six women who have had pre-eclampsia will get it again in a future pregnancy.

Of women who had severe pre-eclampsia, or eclampsia:
- one in two women will get pre-eclampsia in a future pregnancy if their baby needed to be born before 28 weeks of pregnancy
- one in four women will get pre-eclampsia in a future pregnancy if their baby needed to be born before 34 weeks of pregnancy

You should be given information about the chance, in your individual situation, of getting pre-eclampsia in a future pregnancy and about any additional care that you may need. It is advisable to contact your midwife as early as possible once you know you are pregnant again.

**Reproduced from: Royal College of Obstetricians and Gynaecologists. Pre eclampsia patient information leaflet, London, RCOG, Aug 2012, with the permission of the Royal College of Obstetricians and Gynaecologists**

*i4U*

*October 20......*

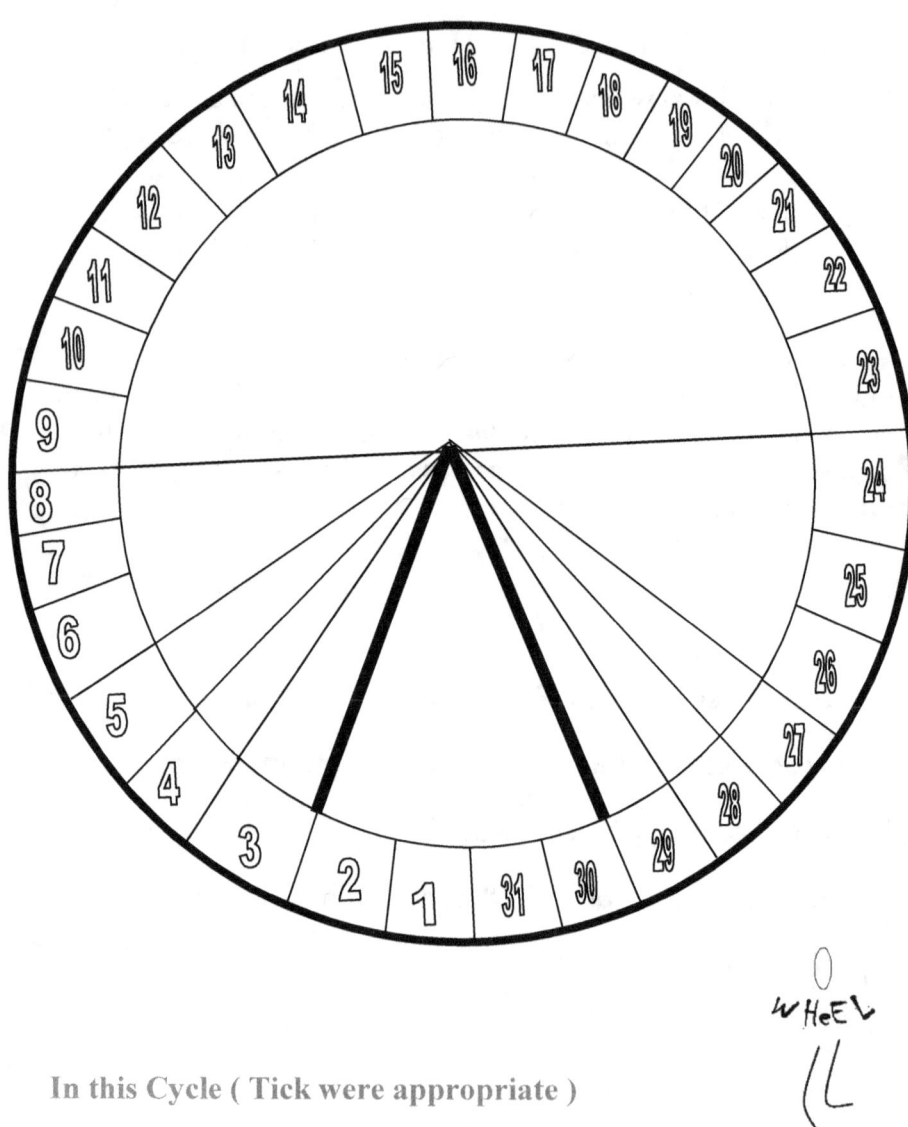

In this Cycle ( Tick were appropriate )

1) Period lasted longer than seven days     YES... NO...
2) Used more pads than is usual for me     YES... NO...
3) Used more tampons than is usual     YES... NO...

| | |
|---|---|
| 4) I Missed School | YES… NO… |
| 5) More pads soaked than is usual | YES… NO… |
| 6) More tampons soaked than is usual | YES… NO… |
| 7) Bleeding with Clots | YES… NO… |
| 8) Heart beating too Fast | YES… NO… |
| 9) Having Heart Palpitation | YES… NO… |
| 10) My Friends say I am Aneamic | YES… NO… |
| 11) Having Blackouts | YES… NO… |
| 12) This Period came too soon | YES…. NO… |
| 13) Getting Tired easily | YES…NO… |
| 14) My HB is less than 8 g/dl | YES…NO… |
| 15) I Missed my Period | YES…NO… |

16) WRITE OTHER COMPLAINTS YOU EXPERIENCED WHICH ARE NOT LISTED ABOVE

If you answered YES to any of the statements above, you probably lost too much blood in this cycle. It is recommended you see your doctor for check ups.

Before you go, Record the number of Pads or Tampons used in this Cycle in the Table below:

| Day of | # of Standard | Or Number of Tampons used | # Improvised Pads used |
|---|---|---|---|
| | | | |

| Menses | Pads used | | |
|---|---|---|---|
| | SOAKED (x) | NOT SOAKED (y) | |
| Day 1 | | | |
| Day 2 | | | |
| Day 3 | | | |
| Day 4 | | | |
| Day 5 | | | |
| Day 6 | | | |
| Day 7 | | | |
| | | | |
| | Total: | Total : | |
| | | | |

Which of the Following Complaints did you experience 7 to 10 days before your menses?

    1) Breast PAIN     YES/ NO
    2) Vomiting     YES/NO
    3) NAUSEA     YES/NO
    4) HEADACHE     YES/NO
    5) DEPRESSION or Feeling Low     YES/NO

6) LOSS OF APPETITE — YES/NO
7) CONSTIPATION — YES/NO
8) BACKACHE — YES/NO
9) ANGER — YES/NO
10) IRRITABLE — YES/NO
11) AGITATION — YES/NO
12) LACK OF SELF CONTROL — YES/NO
13) DIFFICULTIES with concentration — YES/NO
14) TIREDNESS — YES/NO
15) INSOMNIA — YES/NO
16) I FEEL LUMPS IN MY BREASTS — YES/NO
17) WRITE OTHER COMPLAINTS YOU MAY EXPERIENCE WHICH ARE NOT LISTED ABOVE

If you answered YES to most of these statements, you probably experienced pre Menstrual tension or could be suffering from pre menstrual syndrome. Consult your gyneacologist for advice. See a Surgeon or Nurse for advice on Lumps in Your Breast.

*i4U*

*i4U – Information for you*

## Your baby's Movements in Pregnancy

### About this information

This information is for you if you would like to know about your baby's movements during pregnancy. It may also be helpful if you are concerned that your baby has not been moving as much as usual or if you feel that your baby's movements have changed.

It tells you about:

- ✓ what are normal movements for an unborn baby
- ✓ what affects how much you feel your baby move
- ✓ what you should do if your baby's movements are reduced or changed
- ✓ what care you will have if your baby's movements are reduced or changed.

This information aims to help you and your healthcare team make the best decisions about your care. It is not meant to replace advice from a doctor or midwife about your own situation.

### What are normal movements for an unborn baby in pregnancy?

Most women are first aware of their baby moving when they are 18–20 weeks pregnant. However, if this is your first pregnancy, you may not become aware of movements until you are more than 20 weeks pregnant. If you have been pregnant before, you may feel movements as early as 16 weeks. Pregnant women feel their unborn baby's movements as a kick, flutter, swish or roll.

As your baby develops, both the number and type of movements will change with your baby's activity pattern. Usually, afternoon and evening periods are times of peak activity for your baby. During both day and night, your baby has sleep periods that mostly last between 20 and 40 minutes, and are rarely longer than 90 minutes. Your baby will usually not move during these sleep periods.

The number of movements tends to increase until 32 weeks of pregnancy and then stay about the same, although the type of movement may change as you get nearer to your due date. Often, if you are busy, you may not notice all of these movements. Importantly, you should continue to feel your baby move right up to the time you go into labour. Your baby should move during labour too.

## Why are my unborn baby's movements important?

During your pregnancy, feeling your baby move gives you reassurance of his or her wellbeing.

If you notice your baby is moving less than usual or if you have noticed a change in the pattern of movements, it may be the first sign that your baby is unwell and therefore it is essential that you contact your midwife or local maternity unit immediately so that your baby's wellbeing can be assessed.

## How many movements are enough?

There is no specific number of movements which is normal. During your pregnancy, you need to be aware of *your* baby's individual pattern of movements. A reduction or a change in *your* baby's movements is what is important.

## What factors can affect me feeling my baby move?

You are less likely to be aware of your baby's movements when you are active or busy.

If your placenta (afterbirth) is at the front of your uterus (womb), it may not be so easy for you to feel your baby's movements.

Your baby lying head down or bottom first will not affect whether you can feel it move. If your baby's back is lying at the front of your uterus, you may feel fewer movements than if his or her back is lying alongside your own back.

## What can cause my baby to move less?

Certain drugs such as strong pain relief or sedatives can get into an unborn baby's circulation and can make your baby move less. Alcohol and smoking may also affect your baby's movements.

In some cases, a baby may move less because he or she is unwell. Rarely, a baby may have a condition affecting the muscles or nerves that causes him or her to move very little or not at all.

### Should I use a chart to count my baby's movements?

There is not enough evidence to recommend the routine use of a movement chart. It is more important for you to be aware of your baby's individual pattern of movements throughout your pregnancy and you should seek immediate help if you feel that the movements are reduced.

### What if I am unsure about my baby's movements?

If you are unsure whether or not your baby's movements are reduced, you should lie down on your left side and focus on your baby's movements for the next 2 hours. If you do not feel ten or more separate movements during these 2 hours, you should take action (see below).

### What should I do if I feel my baby's movements are reduced or changed?

Always seek professional help immediately. Never go to sleep ignoring a reduction in your baby's movements. Do not rely on any home kits you may have for listening to your baby's heartbeat.

The care you will be given will depend on the stage of your pregnancy:

**Less than 24 weeks pregnant** Most women first become aware of their baby moving when they are 18–20 weeks pregnant. If by 24 weeks you have never felt your baby move, you should contact your midwife, who will check your baby's heartbeat. An ultrasound scan may be arranged and you may be referred to a specialist fetal medicine centre to check your baby's wellbeing.

**Between 24 weeks and 28 weeks pregnant** You should contact your midwife, who will check your baby's heartbeat. You will have a full antenatal check-up that includes checking the size of your uterus, measuring your blood pressure and testing your urine for protein. If your uterus measures smaller than expected, an ultrasound scan may be arranged to check on your baby's growth and development

**Over 28 weeks pregnant** You must contact your midwife or local maternity unit immediately. You *must not* wait until the next day to seek help.

> You will be asked about your baby's movements. You will have a full antenatal check-up, including checking your baby's heartbeat.
>
> Your baby's heart rate will be monitored, usually for at least 20 minutes. This should give you reassurance about your baby's wellbeing. You should be able to see your baby's heart rate increase as he or she moves. You will usually be able to go home once you are reassured.
>
> An ultrasound scan to check on the growth of your baby, as well as the amount of amniotic fluid around your baby, may be arranged *if*:
>
> your uterus measures smaller than expected
>
> your pregnancy has risk factors associated with stillbirth

the heart-rate monitoring is normal but you still feel that your baby's movements are less than usual.

The scan is normally performed within 24 hours of being requested.

These investigations usually provide reassurance that all is well. Most women who experience one episode of reduction in their baby's movements have a straightforward pregnancy and go on to deliver a healthy baby.

If there are any concerns about your baby, your doctor and midwife will discuss this with you. Follow-up scans may be arranged. In some circumstances, you may be advised that it would be safer for your baby to be born as soon as possible. This would depend on your individual situation and how far you are in your pregnancy.

**What should I do if I find my baby's movements are reduced again?**

When you go home you will be advised to keep an eye on your baby's movements and, should your baby have another episode of reduced movements, you must again contact your local maternity unit immediately. Never hesitate to contact your midwife or local maternity unit for advice, no matter how many times this happens.

i4U

Reproduced from: Royal College of Obstetricians and Gynaecologists. Your baby's movements in pregnancy patient information leaflet, London, RCOG, Aug 2012, with the permission of the Royal College of Obstetricians and Gynaecologists

## November 20......

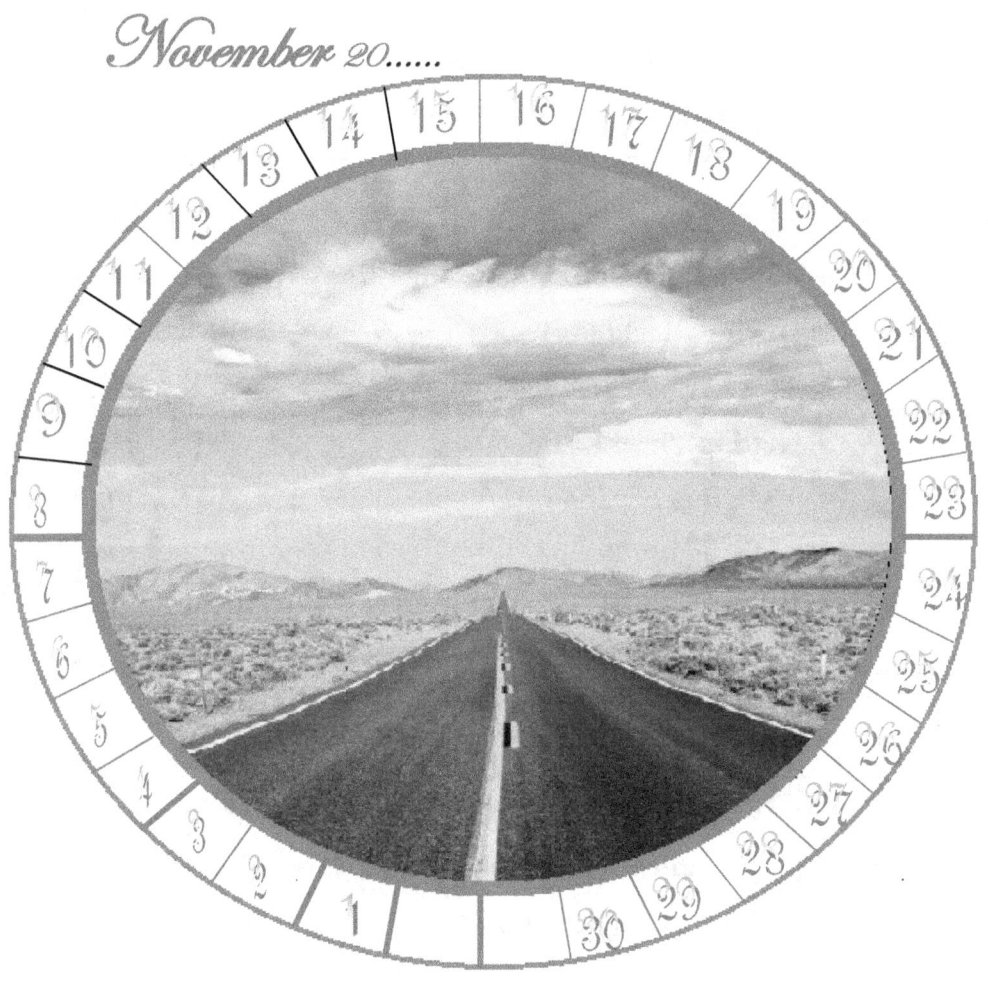

In this Cycle ( Tick were appropriate )

1) Period lasted longer than seven days     YES… NO...
2) Used more pads than is usual for me     YES… NO…
3) Used more tampons than is usual     YES… NO…

4) I missed my Exams                              YES... NO...
5) More pads soaked than is usual                 YES... NO...
6) More tampons soaked than is usual              YES... NO...
7) Bleeding with Clots                            YES... NO...
8) Heart beating too Fast                         YES... NO...
9) Having Heart Palpitations                      YES... NO...
10) I am taking Iron tablets to boost my Hb       YES... NO ...
11) Having Blackouts                              YES... NO...
12) This Period came too soon                     YES.... NO...
13) Getting Tired easily                          YES...NO...
14) My HB is less than 7 g/dl                     YES...NO...
15) I Missed my Period                            YES...NO...
16) **WRITE OTHER COMPLAINTS YOU MAY EXPERIENCE WHICH ARE NOT LISTED ABOVE**

If you answered YES to any of the statements above, you probably lost too much blood in this cycle. It is recommended you see your doctor for check ups.

Before you go, Record the number of Pads or Tampons used in this Cycle in the Table below:

| Day | # of Standard | Or Number of Tampons used | # Improvised Pads used |
|-----|---------------|---------------------------|------------------------|
|     |               |                           |                        |

| Menses | Pads used | | |
|---|---|---|---|
| | SOAKED (x) | NOT SOAKED (y) | |
| Day 1 | | | |
| Day 2 | | | |
| Day 3 | | | |
| Day 4 | | | |
| Day 5 | | | |
| Day 6 | | | |
| Day 7 | | | |
| | | | |
| | Total: | Total : | |
| | | | |

Which of the Following Complaints did you experience 7 to 10 days before your menses?

    1) Breast PAIN                               YES/ NO

    2) Vomiting                                    YES/NO

    3) NAUSEA                                    YES/NO

4) HEADACHE                                    YES/NO
5) DEPRESSION or Feeling Low Spirited          YES/NO
6) LOSS OF APPETITE                            YES/NO
7) CONSTIPATION                                YES/NO
8) BACKACHE                                    YES/NO
9) ANGER                                       YES/NO
10) IRRITABLE                                  YES/NO
11) AGITATION                                  YES/NO
12) LACK OF SELF CONTROL                       YES/NO
13) DIFFICULTIES with concentration            YES/NO
14) TIREDNESS                                  YES/NO
15) INSOMNIA                                   YES/NO
16) I FEEL LUMPS IN MY BREASTS                 YES/NO
17) WRITE OTHER COMPLAINTS YOU MAY EXPERIENCE WHICH ARE NOT LISTED ABOVE

If you answered YES to most of these statements, you probably experienced pre Menstrual tension or could be suffering from pre menstrual syndrome. Consult your gyneacologist for advice. See a Surgeon or Nurse for advice on Lumps in Your Breast.

*i4U - Information for you*

## Treatment for symptoms of the Menopause

### About this information

This information is for you if you are considering treatment for symptoms of the menopause. It tells you about the available treatment options. It may also be helpful if you are a relative or friend of someone who wishes to have treatment for the symptoms of the menopause.

This information does not cover everything you may wish to know about the menopause.

### What is the menopause?

The menopause is when you stop having your periods. It happens when your ovaries stop releasing eggs or your ovaries have been removed and the amount of estrogen hormone in your body falls. Most women in the UK have their menopause between the ages of 45 and 55 years, with the average age being 51 years.

### Key points

> ➢ The menopause is when you stop having your periods.

> ➢ If menopause happens before the age of 40 years, it is called premature menopause or premature ovarian insufficiency.

> Treatment options for the symptoms of the menopause include lifestyle changes, hormone replacement therapy (HRT) and alternative therapies.

> If you wish to consider treatment, your healthcare professional should discuss the benefits and risks of all the available options.

Menopause can occur earlier in some women. If it occurs before the age of 40 years, it is known as premature menopause or premature ovarian insufficiency.

The time before your last period, when your estrogen levels are falling, is called the perimenopause. This can last from a few months to several years. Around half of all women notice physical and/or emotional symptoms during this time.

The most common symptoms are:

- hot flushes
- night sweats
- vaginal dryness
- low mood and/or feeling anxious
- joint and muscle pain
- loss of interest in having sex.

Every woman experiences the menopause differently. Some experience one or two symptoms, which may be mild, while others have more severe and distressing symptoms. Some women choose to go through the menopause without treatment, while others prefer some form of treatment to manage their symptoms, by using either hormone replacement therapy (HRT) or an alternative treatment.

**Do I need any hormone tests before I can start treatment?**

If you have symptoms of the menopause and are over 45 years of age, you will not usually need any hormone tests to diagnose menopause. Treatment options are offered based on your symptoms alone.

**What are my options for the treatment of menopausal symptoms?**

Treatment options for menopausal symptoms include lifestyle changes, non-prescribed treatments and prescribed treatments.

**Lifestyle changes**

Regular aerobic exercise, such as running and swimming, may help, as may low-intensity exercise, such as yoga. Reducing your intake of caffeine and alcohol may also help to reduce hot flushes and night sweats.

**Non-prescribed treatments**

Not every woman chooses HRT for menopausal symptoms. This may be because of your own or family history, or because you have concerns about the safety or side effects of HRT. Treatment options available without prescription are discussed in this section.

**Herbal medicines**

Plants or plant extracts, such as St John's wort, black cohosh and isoflavones (soya products), can help reduce hot flushes and night sweats for some women. However, their safety is unknown and they can react with other medicines that you may be taking for conditions such as breast cancer, epilepsy, heart disease or asthma. You should check with your healthcare professional before taking any herbal medicine.

Unlike conventional medicine, there is no legal obligation for herbal medicines to be licensed. Unlicensed products may vary greatly in their actual contents.

If you buy herbal products, look for a product licence or Traditional Herbal Registration (THR) number on the label (see image) to ensure that what you are buying has been checked for purity. It is advisable to buy remedies from a reputable source.

### Alternative therapy

Alternative therapies such as acupressure, acupuncture or homeopathy may help some women. More research is, however, required on the benefits from these therapies and, if they are used, this should be done with advice from qualified professionals.

### Complementary therapy

You may wish to try a complementary therapy, such as aromatherapy, although the effects of these therapies specifically on your menopausal symptoms are not well known.

### Bioidentical hormones

Commercially available 'bioidentical' hormones are not regulated or licensed in the UK owing to lack of evidence that they are effective or safe to use.

### Prescribed treatments

#### Hormone replacement therapy (HRT)
See the information on HRT below.

#### Non-hormonal medical treatment
Non-hormonal medical treatments, which would need to be prescribed by your doctor, include clonidine or gabapentin for hot flushes.

#### Psychological treatments
Cognitive behavioural therapy (CBT) is a type of psychological treatment. You may be offered CBT for low mood or anxiety related to menopause.

#### Hormone replacement therapy (HRT)
HRT is the most common form of prescribed treatment for menopausal symptoms. It helps to replace the hormone estrogen in your body, which decreases around your menopause. You may sometimes also need other hormones (such as progestogen and testosterone) that your body is no longer producing.

If you are interested in taking HRT, your healthcare professional should discuss the benefits and risks with you before you start the treatment. This discussion should cover both the short-term (over the next 5 years) and the longer term (beyond the next 5 years) benefits and risks for you.

You should also be informed about available alternatives to HRT along with their benefits and risks.

**What are the different types of HRT?**

The type of HRT that you are prescribed depends on your individual situation. If you have a uterus (womb) then a combination of estrogen and progestogen HRT (combined HRT) would be recommended.

Estrogen alone can cause abnormal thickening of the lining of your uterus, which can lead to bleeding. Adding progestogen will prevent this. Progestogen may be given in the form of tablets, patches or a hormone-containing coil.

If combined HRT is started before you have the menopause or within 12 months of your last period then you will be offered a 'cyclical' combined HRT, which should give you regular monthly withdrawal bleeds.

If you start combined HRT more than 12 months after your last period, you may be offered 'continuous' combined HRT (bleed-free HRT). You may experience some vaginal bleeding in the first 3 months, but after this it should stop.

If you have had a hysterectomy then you will be offered estrogen-only HRT.

Women who notice a low sex drive after the menopause may be offered another hormone called testosterone. This is a hormone linked to sex drive in both men and women.

HRT is available as oral tablets, skin patches, injections, body gel or spray, or vaginal ring, cream or pessary.

**Is HRT safe and does it work?**

The effects of HRT have been studied worldwide and research shows that, for most women, HRT works and is safe.

### What are the benefits of HRT?

- It is an effective treatment for hot flushes and low mood associated with the menopause.

- It can improve sexual desire and reduce vaginal dryness.

- It helps keep your bones strong by preventing osteoporosis.

### What are the risks of HRT?

- HRT with estrogen alone (used for women who have no uterus) is associated with little or no increased risk of breast cancer.

- HRT with estrogen and progestogen can increase your risk of breast cancer. This risk is higher the longer you stay on it and reduces when you stop HRT.

- Your individual risk of developing breast cancer depends on underlying risk factors, such as your body weight and your drinking and smoking habits.

- HRT taken as a tablet increases your risk of developing a blood clot, which is not the case if HRT is taken as a patch or gel.

HRT in tablet form slightly increases your risk of stroke, although the overall risk of stroke is very low if you are under the age of 60 years.

Your healthcare professional should discuss your individual risks based on the research evidence at your consultation.

### Can I still have HRT if I have had breast cancer or clots in my legs or lungs?

HRT may still be an option for you and you should discuss this with your healthcare professional, who may seek advice or refer you to a menopause specialist.

### Can I take HRT if I have diabetes or high blood pressure?

HRT should not affect your blood sugar control. If you are diabetic or have very high blood pressure, your healthcare professional may consult with a specialist before prescribing HRT.

### Would taking HRT prevent dementia?

It is not known whether HRT affects the development of dementia.

### Do I still need to use contraception when taking HRT?

HRT does not provide contraception. You need to continue using contraception for 1 year after your last period if this happens after the age of 50 years. If your last period happens before you are 50 years of age then you need to continue using contraception for 2 years.

### When should I seek advice after starting HRT?

You should have a review appointment with your healthcare professional after 3 months of starting or changing HRT, and then yearly thereafter if all remains well.

You may notice some vaginal bleeding in the first 3 months of starting or changing HRT, but if you experience any bleeding after 3 months then you should see your healthcare professional straight away.

### How long can I take HRT for?

There are no set time limits for how long you can be on HRT. The benefits and risks of taking HRT will depend on your individual situation, and your healthcare professional should discuss these with you.

### How do I stop HRT?

You can stop your HRT suddenly or reduce gradually before stopping it. The chances of your symptoms coming back is the same either way.

### Do I need a referral to a menopause specialist?

If your menopausal symptoms are not responding to HRT or there are reasons why HRT may not be considered safe for you, your healthcare professional may seek advice from, or refer you to, a menopause specialist.

### Which treatment is best for my hot flushes and night sweats?

If you are troubled with hot flushes and night sweats, you should be offered HRT after discussing its benefits and risks. You may wish to discuss the alternative options described above with your healthcare professional.

### Which treatment is best for my low mood?

HRT is an effective treatment for low mood. CBT is also helpful in treating low mood and anxiety related to the menopause.

Low mood as a result of the menopause is different from depression. Antidepressants are not helpful unless you have been diagnosed with depression. If you are on antidepressants, it is safe to take HRT as well as use CBT.

### Which treatment is best for my lack of interest in sex?

HRT containing estrogen and/or progestogen may be helpful as treatment for low sexual desire during menopause. If this doesn't work then you should talk to your healthcare professional about whether to consider another hormone called testosterone, which is linked to sex drive in both men and women.

### Which treatment is best for my vaginal dryness?

Many women find using vaginal moisturisers and lubricants helpful for vaginal dryness. Ask your healthcare professional about the best one for you.

Estrogen given vaginally in the form of a tablet, cream or ring is effective in treating vaginal dryness. Low-dose vaginal estrogens can be used for as long as you need to and can also be safely used in combination with HRT. These can also reduce bladder infections and help urinary symptoms. If you experience any unexpected vaginal bleeding, you should tell your healthcare professional. Other forms of HRT can also help with vaginal dryness.

### What is premature menopause (premature ovarian insufficiency) and what causes it?

This is when you go through the menopause before the age of 40 years. Usually, no cause is found for this. It can be caused by surgery on the ovaries, chemotherapy, or radiotherapy to the pelvis. It can also run in families. Other less common causes include chromosomal problems, such as Turner syndrome, and autoimmune disease when the body's immune system attacks the developing eggs.

### How is premature menopause diagnosed?

If your periods become infrequent or stop before the age of 40 years and/or you experience menopausal symptoms, you should see your healthcare professional. You will be offered blood tests to measure your hormone levels to help diagnose premature menopause. The diagnosis is made after two blood tests are performed 4–6 weeks apart.

### Are there any health risks related to premature menopause?

You are likely to notice the symptoms of menopause, such as hot flushes and mood changes. There is also an increased risk of developing osteoporosis and cardiac disease in later life. Osteoporosis can lead to broken bones if not treated. Premature menopause will affect your fertility, and your chance of getting pregnant will be greatly reduced.

### What is the treatment for premature menopause?

Treatment for premature menopause involves the replacement of hormones in the form of either HRT or the combined oral contraceptive pill. Both are effective in treating hot flushes and keeping your bones strong.

While the combined oral contraceptive pill has the advantage of also providing contraception, HRT is a safer option if you have high blood pressure.

It is important for you to continue the treatment at least until the average age of natural menopause. By taking HRT, you are simply replacing the hormones your body is lacking, and so there are no added risks.

If you are thinking about getting pregnant, you will need a referral to a fertility specialist. Your healthcare professional may also suggest referral to a menopause specialist.

**Reproduced from: Royal College of Obstetricians and Gynaecologists. Treatment for symptoms of the menopause patient information leaflet, London, RCOG, Feb 2018, with the permission of the Royal College of Obstetricians and Gynaecologists**

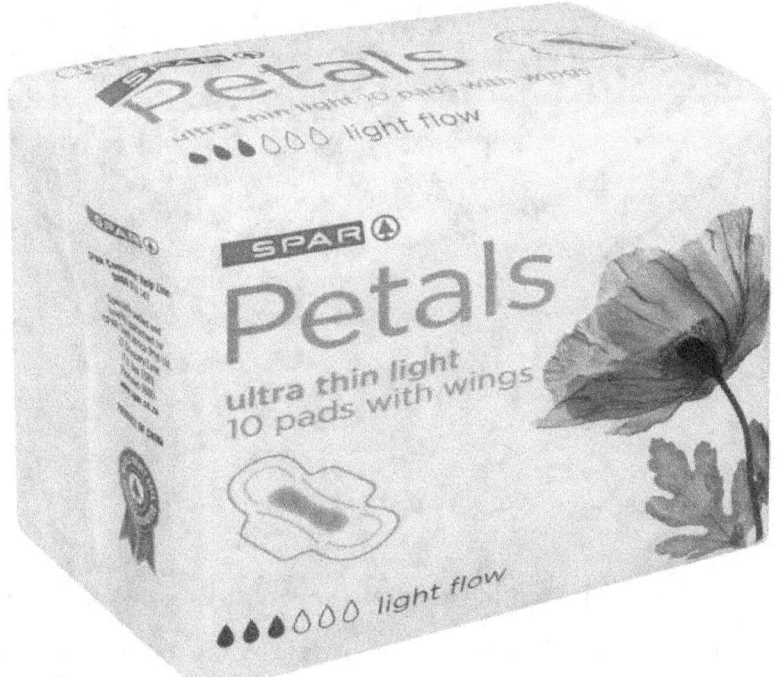

i4U

# December 20......

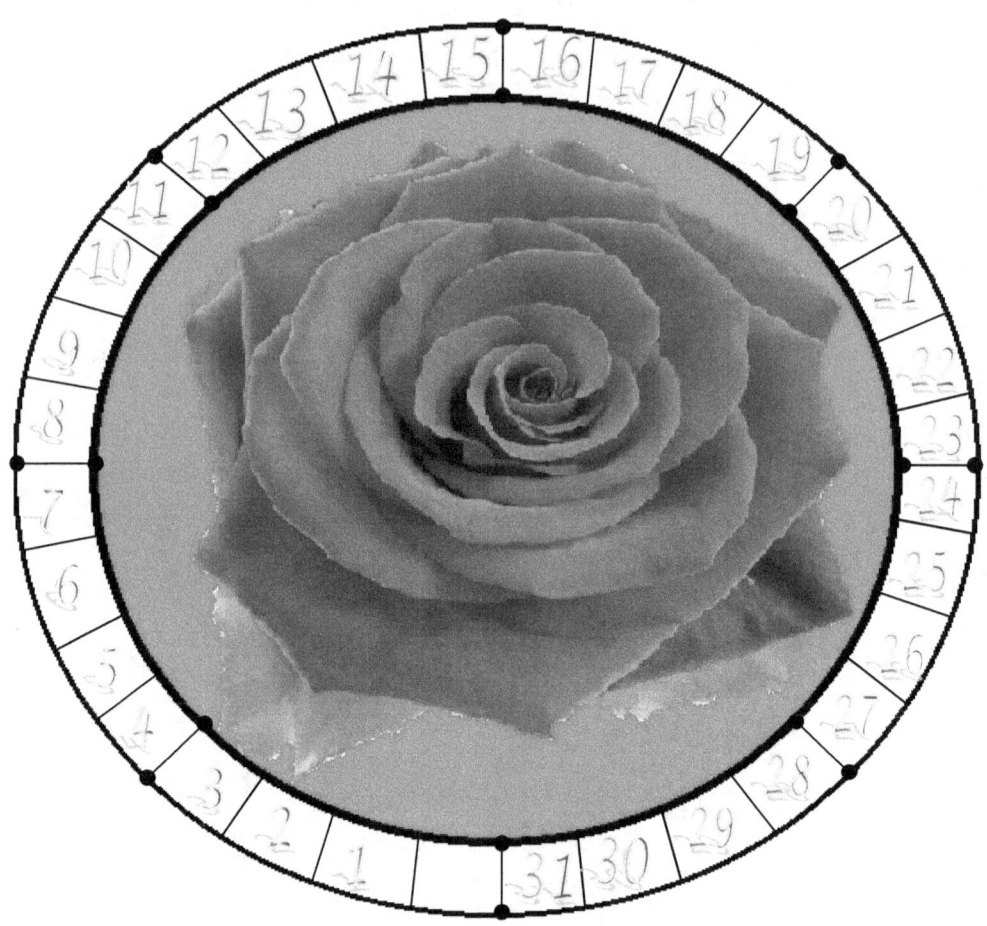

wHeEL

In this Cycle ( Tick were appropriate )

1) Period lasted longer than seven days   YES... NO...
2) Used more pads than is usual for me   YES... NO...
3) Used more tampons than is usual   YES... NO...

4) I had very painful menses — YES… NO…
5) More pads soaked than is usual — YES… NO…
6) More tampons soaked than is usual — YES… NO…
7) Bleeding with Clots — YES… NO…
8) Heart beating too Fast — YES… NO…
9) Used Improvised Pads — YES… NO…
10) Menses made me ill; missed the Exams — YES… NO …
11) My Face & eye lids appears swollen — YES… NO…
12) This Period came too soon — YES…. NO…
13) Getting Tired easily — YES…NO…
14) I think My HB is Low — YES…NO…
15) I Missed my Period — YES…NO…
16) WRITE OTHER COMPLAINTS YOU MAY EXPERIENCE WHICH ARE NOT LISTED ABOVE

If you answered YES to any of the statements above, you probably lost too much blood in this cycle. It is recommended you see your doctor for check ups.

*i4U*

Before you go, Record the number of Pads or Tampons used in this Cycle in the Table below:

| Day of Menses | # of Standard Pads used | Or Number of Tampons used | # Improvised Pads used |
|---|---|---|---|
| | SOAKED (x) | NOT SOAKED (y) | |
| Day 1 | | | |
| Day 2 | | | |
| Day 3 | | | |
| Day 4 | | | |
| Day 5 | | | |
| Day 6 | | | |
| Day 7 | | | |
| | | | |
| | Total: | Total : | |
| | | | |

Which of the Following Complaints did you experience 7 to 10 days before your menses?

1) Breast PAIN — YES/ NO
2) Vomiting — YES/NO
3) NAUSEA — YES/NO
4) HEADACHE — YES/NO
5) DEPRESSION or Feeling Low — YES/NO
6) LOSS OF APPETITE — YES/NO
7) CONSTIPATION — YES/NO
8) BACKACHE — YES/NO
9) ANGER — YES/NO
10) IRRITABLE — YES/NO
11) AGITATION — YES/NO
12) LACK OF SELF CONTROL — YES/NO
13) DIFFICULTIES with concentration — YES/NO
14) TIREDNESS — YES/NO
15) INSOMNIA — YES/NO
16) I FEEL LUMPS IN MY BREASTS — YES/NO
17) WRITE OTHER COMPLAINTS YOU MAY EXPERIENCE WHICH ARE NOT LISTED ABOVE

If you answered yes to most of these statements, you probably experienced pre Menstrual tension or could be suffering from pre menstrual syndrome. Consult your gyneacologist for advice. See a Surgeon or Nurse for advice on Lumps in Your Breast.

*i4U- Information for you*

# Skin conditions of the Vulva

**About this information**

This information is for you if you want to know about skin conditions affecting the vulva. If you are a partner or relative of someone who is in this situation, you may also find this leaflet helpful.

**What is the vulva?**

The vulva is the area surrounding the opening of the vagina. It includes the labia (the inner and outer vaginal lips) and the clitoris.

**What are the symptoms of a Vulval skin condition?**

Many women have symptoms, which can occur at any age. The most common are itching, pain, soreness or a change in the skin colour and texture. These symptoms may be caused by a condition that only affects the vulva, but they can sometimes be a sign of a more general medical problem or other skin disease. Your symptoms may be made worse by moisture, heat or rubbing and by the use of scented products/deodorants.

**Do I need to see a doctor?**

Yes. It is important that you visit your doctor to see what may be causing the problem. He or she should also be able to advise on how to help your symptoms.

**What will happen when I see the doctor?**

Your doctor will ask you questions about the symptoms affecting your vulva and also about any symptoms in other parts of your body. You will also be asked about what medication you are taking and about your personal and family medical history. This is because conditions such as thyroid disease, diabetes, anaemia or a history of hay fever, asthma or eczema can be linked to some vulval skin conditions.

Women can often have an allergic reaction in their vulval skin, so it may be useful to list any treatments such as creams and ointments that you have been using on your skin in that area. Sometimes irritation can also be caused by chemicals in washing powders and bath or sanitary products.

The skin of your vulva will be examined for signs of a skin condition that might affect other parts of your body. Your doctor may look at your mouth, scalp, elbows, knees and nails, the inside of your vagina and the skin around your anus.

Vulval skin conditions may sometimes make sex difficult. This can be very distressing. You may be asked some intimate questions to help reach a diagnosis and to decide which treatment is the most suitable for you.

**Will I need tests?**

If your doctor thinks you may have a more general health problem, you may need to have blood tests and swabs to check for infection.

Often your doctor may be able to decide what is wrong from the appearance of your skin. You will be offered treatment that is most likely to work for your condition. If your skin does not get better or if the diagnosis is unclear, you may be advised to have a biopsy (a tiny sample of skin taken for testing).

Biopsies are often performed in the outpatient clinic, using local anaesthetic to numb the area so you will feel no pain when the biopsy is taken.

Itching of the vulva may be caused by an allergy. You can develop sensitivity after you have been using a product for some time. Your doctor may suggest having further tests to find out what you are sensitive to.

**What conditions might be causing my symptoms?**

There are several skin conditions that may affect the vulva, including:

> - **Lichen sclerosus-**This can affect women of any age but is most often found in women after the menopause. It is thought to be caused by a problem with the immune system. It is not

related to the use of hormonal contraceptives or hormone replacement therapy (HRT).
- **Lichen planus-**This condition tends to cause pain rather than itching. It can affect the skin anywhere on the body, particularly the mouth.
- **Vulval dermatitis (lichen simplex)-**This can happen if you have sensitive skin, dermatitis or eczema. It may also extend to your inner thighs or pubic area. Stress and chemical irritants may make your symptoms worse.
- **Vulval atrophy-**This can happen when the female hormone estrogen falls, usually after the menopause. It causes the skin to be pale and can cause itching or soreness.
- **VIN (vulval intraepithelial neoplasia)-**VIN is found in the vulva and can only be diagnosed by taking a biopsy. In this condition there are changes in the skin that may become cancerous over time. It is similar to the pre-cancerous changes that are looked for in cervical smears. Your doctor may advise you to have your cervix and vagina examined in detail with a microscopic camera (colposcopy) to check those areas as well. Women who have lichen sclerosus may sometimes have VIN.
- **Candida infection (thrush)-**This tends to cause irritation and soreness of the vulva rather than the discharge that most women are aware of when it affects the vagina. Sometimes candida can be passed to a sexual partner so it is important that they are checked and treated if necessary, if your symptoms don't improve.

> **Psoriasis-**This may affect the vulva and cause dryness and thickening of the skin. Other parts of your body such as the nails and scalp may also be affected.

Apart from candida, the above conditions are not infectious and will not be passed to a sexual partner.

## What treatments might I have?

Most symptoms respond to simple measures, such as avoiding irritants, using a soap substitute for cleansing and making sure the skin is moisturised, but sometimes treatment is needed. The type of treatment will depend on which skin condition you have.

Medication such as antihistamines or anti-itching drugs may help, especially if you are having difficulty sleeping.

If you have lichen sclerosus or lichen planus, you may need to use steroid ointment. This will improve symptoms for most women. Once treatment is completed, the colour and texture of your skin may not return to normal. Women under the age of 50 tend to respond best to these treatments. Unfortunately, symptoms often come back and long-term treatment may be needed.

About 1 in 10 women with lichen sclerosus have symptoms that do not improve with steroids. If this happens, you should be referred to a specialist clinic.

If your skin is pale, which suggests a lack of estrogen, you may be offered a short course of estrogen cream.

Candida is treated with antifungal tablets and creams. If you have candida that keeps coming back, you may need treatment for a longer period, often up to 6 months.

Most conditions of the vulva will be helped by these simple measures. If your symptoms persist despite treatment, it is important to tell your GP, who should refer you to a specialist.

## What if I have VIN?

You will usually have the affected piece of skin removed by surgery. If you don't have this done, the doctor will take several tiny skin samples to make sure there is no cancer present.

Most small areas of VIN can be removed without any problems. If a large area of skin needs to be removed, you may need to have reconstructive (plastic) surgery to prevent excessive scarring, skin tension or problems with sex.

You may be offered other treatments such as laser or creams but these are not suitable for everyone. Your doctor will discuss the best option for you in your situation.

**What follow-up should I have?**

You should check your vulva regularly. You can ask your GP or practice nurse to do this for you but you can also do it yourself. If you examine yourself regularly, you become aware of what is normal for you, and can quickly detect any changes.

If you have lichen sclerosus or lichen planus, you will usually be followed up by your GP rather than at the hospital. It is particularly important with these conditions that you watch out carefully for any change in your symptoms and go back to your doctor if you have any concerns. This is because there is a small risk that skin cancer may develop.

If you have VIN, you will have regular check-ups, usually once a year, at a specialist clinic. This is because there is a higher risk of developing cancer of the vulva. You will also be given advice to look out for ulcers or blisters on the skin. If you develop these or have any concerns, you should tell your doctor so that you can be seen earlier if necessary.4

## Tips for care of the vulva

Vulval skin is very sensitive so it is important to avoid irritants that may make symptoms worse.

## Washing

- ➢ Washing with water and soap may cause dry skin and make itching worse. Using soap substitutes can be soothing and protective, and will stop the skin from becoming as dry and irritated. Aqueous cream (a special type of moisturiser available without prescription from your pharmacy or on prescription from your doctor) can be used instead of soap. It can be kept in the fridge and also be dabbed on to cool and soothe the skin.
- ➢ Too much washing can make the symptoms worse so you should clean the vulval area only once a day. If possible, have a shower rather than a bath, but if you do have a bath it is helpful to add an emollient (see below). Don't use antiseptics. Avoid using sponges or flannels to wash the vulva as these can irritate the skin. To dry, pat the area with a soft towel or use a hairdryer on a cool setting held well away from the skin.
- ➢ Avoid wearing panty liners or sanitary towels on a regular basis. Avoid coloured toilet paper.

## Clothing

- ➢ Wear loose-fitting cotton or silk underwear (rather than synthetic, dyed underwear). White or light-coloured underwear is preferable as dark textile dyes may cause allergies.
- ➢ Avoid clothes such as tights, leggings, tight jeans and cycling shorts. At home, you may find it more comfortable to wear loose-fitting clothes without underwear. Sleep without underwear.
- ➢ Avoid using fabric conditioners and biological washing powders.

## Irritants

- Avoid using soaps, shower gels, scrubs, bubble baths, deodorants, baby wipes and douches as all of these may contain skin irritants.
- Be careful when using over-the-counter preparations as some of those available may aggravate allergies and prolong symptoms, e.g. baby or nappy creams, herbal creams (tea tree oil, aloe vera) and thrush treatments.
- If you tend to scratch your skin, keep your nails trimmed if possible and avoid wearing nail polish.

## Emollients

Emollients (moisturising creams and ointments) help protect the skin. They are available over the counter or on prescription. Using a moisturiser even when you do not have symptoms can prevent flare-ups. It is important to find the one that suits you best – if the first one you try does not relieve your symptoms, it is worth trying a different one.5

**Reproduced from: Royal College of Obstetricians and Gynaecologists. skin Conditions of the vulva patient information leaflet, London, RCOG, Dec 2013, with the permission of the Royal College of Obstetricians and Gynaecologists**

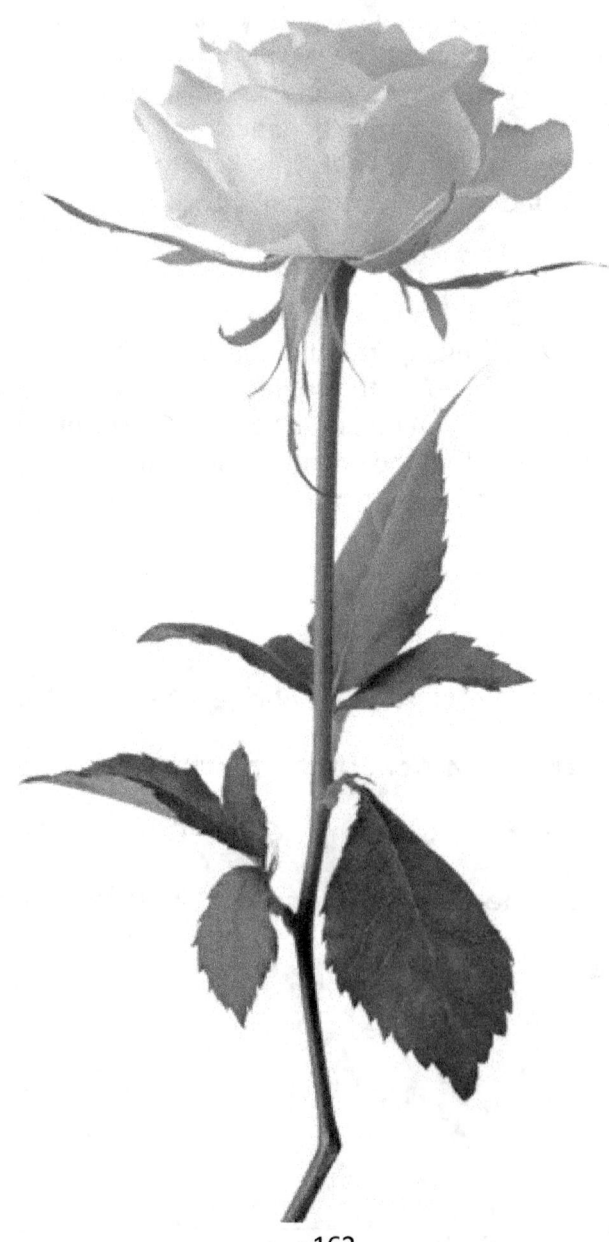

www.ingramcontent.com/pod-product-compliance
Lightning Source LLC
Chambersburg PA
CBHW071543220526
45469CB00003B/898